Reimagining Therapy through Social Contextual Analyses

This book attempts to 'shake up' the current complacency around therapy and 'mental health' behaviours by putting therapy fully into context using Social Contextual Analysis; showing how changes to our social, discursive, and societal environments, rather than changes to an individual's 'mind', will reduce suffering from the 'mental health' behaviours.

Guerin challenges many assumptions about both current therapy and psychology, and offers alternative approaches, synthesized from sociology, social anthropology, sociolinguistics, and elsewhere. The book provides a way of addressing the 'mental health' behaviours including actions, talking, thinking, and emotions, by taking people's external life situations into account, and not relying on an imagined 'internal source'. Guerin describes the broad contexts for current Western therapies, referring to social, discursive, cultural, societal, and economic contexts, and suggests that we need to research the components of therapies and stop treating therapies as units. He reframes different types of therapy away from their abstract jargons, offering an alternative approach grounded in our real social worlds, aligning with new thinking that challenges the traditional methods of therapy, and also providing a better framework for rethinking psychology itself. The book ultimately suggests more emphasis should be put on 'mental health' behaviours as arising from social issues including the modern contexts of extreme capitalism, excessive bureaucracy, weakened discursive communities, and changing forms of social relationships.

Practical guidelines are provided for building the reimagined therapies into clinics and institutions where labelling and pathologizing the 'mental health' behaviours will no longer be needed. By putting 'mental health' behaviours and therapy into a naturalistic or ecological social sciences framework, this book will be practical and fascinating reading for professional therapists, counsellors, social workers, and mental health nurses, as well as academics interested in psychology and the social sciences more generally.

Bernard Guerin has worked in both Australia and New Zealand researching and teaching to merge psychology with the social sciences. His main research now focuses on contextualizing 'mental health' behaviours, working with Indigenous communities, and exploring social contextual analyses especially for language use and thinking.

Exploring the Environmental and Social Foundations of Human Behaviour

Series Editor
Bernard Guerin
Professor of Psychology, University of South Australia

Can you imagine that everything people do, say and think is shaped directly by engaging with our many environmental and social contexts? Humans would then really be part of their environment.

For current psychology, however, people only engage with metaphorical 'internal' environments or brains events, and everything we do somehow originates hidden in there. But what if all that we do and think originated out in our worlds, and what we call 'internal' is merely language and conversations which were also shaped by engaging in our external discursive, cultural and societal environments?

Exploring the Environmental and Social Foundations of Human Behaviour is an exciting new book series about developing the next generation of ways to understand what people do, say and think. Human behaviour is shaped through directly engaging in our diverse contexts of resources, social relationships, economics, culture, discourses, colonization, patriarchy, society, and the opportunities afforded by our birth contexts. Even language and thinking arise from our external social and discursive contexts, and so the 'internal' and brain metaphors will disappear as psychology becomes merged with the social sciences.

The series is therefore a-disciplinary and presents analyses or contextually-engaged research on topics which describe or demonstrate how human behaviour arises from direct engagement with the worlds in which we are embedded.

In this series:

How to Rethink Psychology: New Metaphors for Understanding People and their Behavior: Volume 1

How to Rethink Human Behavior: A Practical Guide to Social Contextual Analysis: Volume 2

How to Rethink Mental Illness: The Human Contexts Behind the Labels: Volume 3

Turning Psychology into Social Contextual Analysis: Volume 4

Turning Psychology into a Social Science: Volume 5

Turning Mental Health into Social Action: Volume 6

Reimagining Therapy through Social Contextual Analyses: Finding New Ways to Support People in Distress: Volume 7

Reimagining Therapy through Social Contextual Analyses

Finding New Ways to Support People in Distress

Bernard Guerin

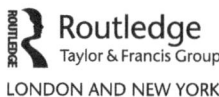
Routledge
Taylor & Francis Group

LONDON AND NEW YORK

Cover image: Getty Images

First published 2023
by Routledge
4 Park Square, Milton Park, Abingdon, Oxon OX14 4RN

and by Routledge
605 Third Avenue, New York, NY 10158

Routledge is an imprint of the Taylor & Francis Group, an informa business

© 2023 Bernard Guerin

The right of Bernard Guerin to be identified as author of this work has been
asserted in accordance with sections 77 and 78 of the Copyright, Designs and
Patents Act 1988.

All rights reserved. No part of this book may be reprinted or reproduced or
utilised in any form or by any electronic, mechanical, or other means, now
known or hereafter invented, including photocopying and recording, or in
any information storage or retrieval system, without permission in writing
from the publishers.

Trademark notice: Product or corporate names may be trademarks or registered
trademarks, and are used only for identification and explanation without
intent to infringe.

British Library Cataloguing-in-Publication Data
A catalogue record for this book is available from the British Library

Library of Congress Cataloging-in-Publication Data
A catalog record has been requested for this book

ISBN: 978-1-032-29243-4 (hbk)
ISBN: 978-1-032-29240-3 (pbk)
ISBN: 978-1-003-30057-1 (ebk)

DOI: 10.4324/9781003300571

Typeset in Bembo
by Taylor & Francis Books

Contents

PART 3
Rethinking 'mental health' as living in restrictive bad life situations

Illustrations

Figures

Tables

Boxes

Preface

This book is a detailed and critical look at 'therapy'. For reasons given in Chapter 1, it looks at both 'therapy' and 'mental health' in relation to the person's life contexts, rather than misattributing cause to something 'inside' or 'internal' to the person. This produces a very original and forward-looking approach.

For this book I have read masses of academic and non-academic books of all sorts of approaches said to be 'therapeutic'. Mainstream and non-mainstream. I watched a lot of videos of all such 'therapies' and participated in a number of workshops of different kinds. I talked with many therapists. As will become clear, I distrust the words of therapists about what they do but trust their descriptions of what goes on.

My main conclusions from all this are many, outlined in the last two chapters: language is the basis for most therapies; most therapies are somewhat effective but not for the reasons they present in their theories and marketing; the language of talking *about* therapy is a complete mishmash of abstract and topsy-turvy discourses; such discourses also seem to help some people in some ways *despite* being fanciful; the biggest fault of almost all current therapies is not attempting to help the person with their actual life situations, which are shaping all the problems encountered. This latter is made more difficult for therapists because of restrictions enforced through professional and governmental agencies.

Despite all this, I come away with great hope for a new version of therapy, in which there is never a single therapist, and the person and the 'therapists' work towards improving the person's life situation as well as improving how they talk about themselves and their life (what currently goes on in therapy) and improving how the people around them respond to such talk (improving their discursive communities in life). The new 'experts' are not experts of some disembodied mind 'inside' the person, but experts on how people adapt to bad life situations and how to 'fix the life situation' rather than trying to 'fix the person' through talking. This requires a serious reimagining of what therapy must become.

Acknowledgments

I will start by thanking Brandon Umphrey who wrote to me a long time ago and wondered if I had ever collected everything about my contextual approaches that might change the way we do therapy. I had not done this, but that made me begin and this is the first result.

I want to thank Matt, Rory, and Berny for allowing me to see how they work in alternative ways in therapy. I am suggesting things they might not agree with, but much of it stems from my observations through them. I also thank Mel Beaton for allowing me to use the figures from her Honours thesis in Chapter 9.

I thank all the students, both undergraduate and my wonderful graduate students, who allowed me to rehearse and develop many of these thoughts in discussions (Kate, Adan, Millie, Kris, Eden, Scarlett, Nikia, and others). Often I was wildly extemporizing, in full flight over a beer; but this pushed me to always take these ideas further and further. That they listened, helped me to develop and critically extend the ideas contained in this book. There is more to come, especially their case studies illustrating these ideas in practice.

As always, a big thanks to Eleanor and Alex for their faith in this book series, and for seeing me through the whole production process so calmly and professionally.

Part 1
Dissecting current therapies

Part 1

Observing correct therapies

1 Psychology, pop psychology, and common-sense psychology

Whatever were they thinking for 150 years?

Many of the problems with therapy come from problematic ideas of 'why people do what they do'. There is a standard everyday version of 'why people do what they do', which psychology has assumed to be correct and has therefore spent 150 years trying to explain and predict using that lay model. Many, like me, however, think that particular model of human behaviour is wrong and is just a prop to get on with everyday life, rather than an accurate description needing to be explained (albeit useful in everyday life).

The basic problem is that when people cannot see an obvious or salient 'cause' for the way a human behaves, they attribute the 'cause' to an abstract series of words (cf. Edwards & Potter, 1993). These words can be about an 'inner' person or 'inner' experience, a personality causing behaviours, abstract 'cognitive processes', 'inner' unconscious and conscious desires and urges, instincts, mind, mental, brain processes (abstract when used as a 'cause'), decision-making centres, or a plethora of other abstract 'causes' such as self-esteem, intelligence, etc. When in real doubt, people and psychologists have resorted to using 'meaning', 'perceived', and 'psychological' as backups. Or when the behaviours are painful or unwanted, the 'internal' attributed 'cause' then becomes a 'disease', 'mental illness', 'disorder', or even more abstract words ('borderline personality disorder'!).

As discourses, all the words and phrases above function in conversation to appear 'as if' they explain something, but they actually hedge any responsibility or import by being abstract, unobservable, and vague. In everyday life they function fine usually, since knowing the 'real' cause is never the issue; the words are being used to affect listeners to work our social lives. But psychology has had 150 years of problems because it has seen its task as that of explaining these everyday abstract ideas, which were originated for a very different function than accurate observation and explanation.

This has led to 150 years of serially changing one set of abstract words for a new set and believing that progress has been made, as Figure 1.1 suggests. For example, currently, instead of therapy changing or controlling unconscious urges, therapy now tries to repair faulty cognitive processes—at least that is how they talk about it. Other groups talk about therapy as repairing the broken brain.

DOI: 10.4324/9781003300571-2

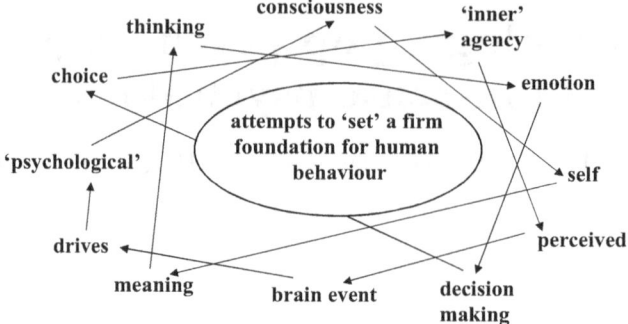

Figure 1.1 Words often used to construct the 'foundations' for human behaviour but which constantly get switched or bounced around uncritically

The real problem for therapy, however, goes further than just this; from that plethora of abstract words, the goal of therapy has been to change or alter what is *purported* to be the causes of painful behaviours, so the goal has actually been *to change these abstract words* which were invented to satisfy everyday conversation. Figure 1.2 tries to illustrate this while Figure 1.3 shows where we are heading in this book.

On the other hand, an advantage of therapists over most academics is that they are usually closely involved with real persons experiencing real suffering, no matter what words they end up using, so they have done more observations and can experiment with ways to change or remove the suffering without necessarily sticking to or following the abstract words.

This fundamental disparity between (1) the observations and actions therapists make in social interaction and (2) their verbal explanations, will follow us through this book. I will repeatedly suggest paying close attention to what therapies have done, at least when they have made good *observations* and have also tried new things out (Pierre Janet was a model here). On the other hand, when therapists go on to *explain* the causes of the suffering or the causes for

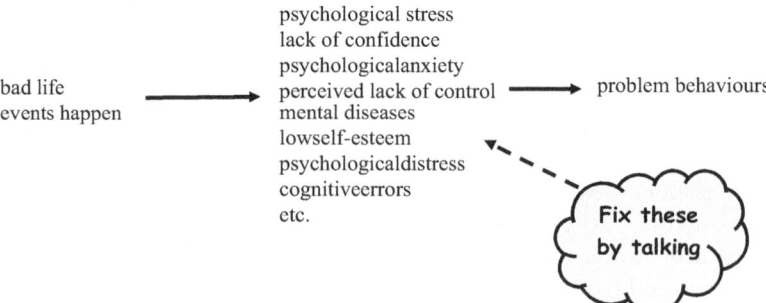

Figure 1.2 'Explanations' and 'therapy' in psychology for 150 years

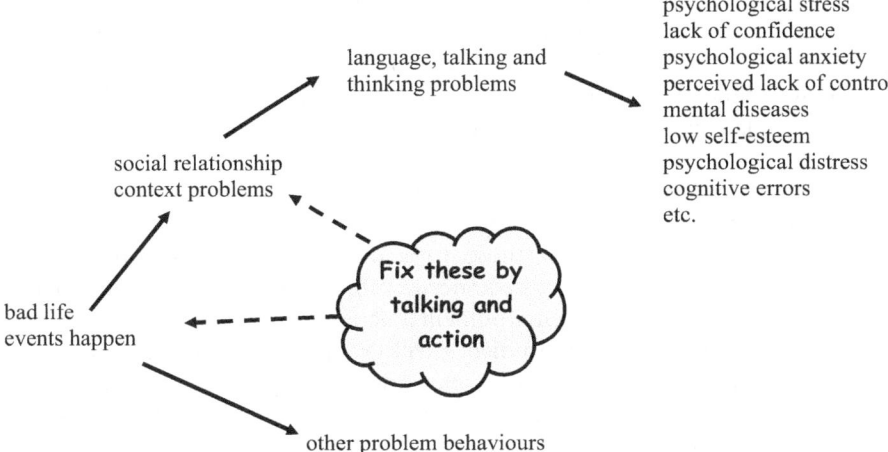

Figure 1.3 Contextual explanations

why what they tried worked, we can mostly ignore this because it gets back to the morass of abstractions. My experience is that most therapies do some good, and I will explore why this might be the case in Chapter 5 when we look at the components of therapies. But their theories for why what they do might work are add-on words based on lay talk for why humans do what they do.

What can we do instead of using abstraction?

There have always been alternative explanations for human behaviour, which do not rely on the everyday discourses of hidden 'inner' causes (misattributions). A few have been within psychology and therapy, but more are to be found within sociology, social anthropology, sociolinguistics, and elsewhere. In the second part of this book, I will use my own synthesis of all these which is *a-disciplinary*, it combines all as one (Guerin, 2016a, 2016b, 2017, 2020a, 2020b, 2020c). This also has an advantage of making what shapes human behaviour much more observable than for any of the abstract theories.

The main point is that when psychologists and others cannot observe a clear or salient 'cause' for human behaviour, *they have not been looking hard enough* or *they have been looking in the wrong place*. What shapes human behaviour is outside of the body, and the skin is not a magical enclosure for some 'inner' person (Bentley, 1941a/1975, 1941b). *There is no 'inner' person looking out;* that is a false metaphor, which has been known for a long time (Hinton, 2016).

As we will discover in Chapters 6 and 7, much of human behaviour is shaped by social, societal, and structural contexts, which are very material, but *which cannot be seen easily.* For example, societies have different patriarchal contexts which shape strong differences between most males and most females (differences in the use of makeup, clothes, etc.), but how this exactly is shaped is difficult to observe, at least with quick or superficial observations, since it occurs over time and through many different people (including media now). Like lay explanations in everyday life, it is easier to invent abstract 'internal' 'causes'.

So, what I call Social Contextual Analyses just brings together what we know from sociology, social anthropology, sociolinguistics, and elsewhere (such as behaviour analysis) to show those parts of our worlds, environments or contexts which shape what we do. Social anthropologists, for example, have focussed more on the natural environmental ecology (food, climate) because of the people they have typically studied: small groups in remote locations living with subsistence economies. Modern humans are shaped more by large and diffuse societal contexts, which are not abstract but very real and backed up by very real police, armies, and laws.

I will do a little introduction to Social Contextual Analyses in Chapters 6 and 7, but I will do this mostly by giving tips about how to observe and analyse what people are doing, and mainly for dealing with 'mental health' behaviours. Chapters 8 and 9 will then show how the 'mental health' behaviours are shaped by our external life worlds and do not originate inside our heads or brains or minds, or abstract 'cognitive processes'. I do not claim to have originated all these ideas but have put them together. (I also do not list all the references because they slow down the reading, but everything I say has a long list of predecessors.)

Appling this to what we call 'mental health' and therapy

We can apply the work of the social sciences and some psychology, then, to reimagining and changing what we currently call 'mental health' to show how those behaviours were shaped by life contexts (Guerin, 2017, 2020c). But the main aim of this book is to look at what is done under the rubric of 'therapy' in its contexts; that is, what are the contexts for doing therapy, the contexts of those seeking therapy, and the outcomes of whatever is done in therapy (Chapters 9 to 11).

One of the main points, once we examine the contexts shaping 'mental health' behaviours and therapies and stop building ever more stories about 'inner' worlds, is the overarching role of language in all of this. Most 'mental health' problems are really 'language problems', once a better contextualized version of using language is given (Chapter 7), but contextually, we will see that 'language problems' are really problems with our social and societal relationships. Even what we call 'emotional' behaviour will be seen to be a result of the reliance on language use in our everyday lives. And therapy itself consists now almost exclusively of talking, although we will see in Chapter 7 that language is not primarily about words, when looked at functionally in context, but is about doing things to social relationships in a specialized way. So 'language disorders' and even 'thinking disorders' are really social and societal relationship disorders.

Putting all this together will produce some surprising and innovative ways of moving forward with what we currently call 'mental health' and 'therapy (Chapters 10 to 12). Box 1.1 gives a few spoilers for this.

Box 1.1 Implications for therapy if you assume that human behaviour originates 'inside' or is shaped by life contexts

Behaviour originates inside a person	**Behaviour is shaped by our contexts**
Assume the everyday idea that behaviour arises from 'within' a person as decisions, brain processes, choices, mind, mental processes, urges, instinct, unconscious, etc.	*Assume that actions, talking and thinking are shaped by our interacting with the many contexts in which we are embedded through our lives: social, societal, economic, cultural, patriarchal, colonizing, etc.*
Any problems require an expert in mind, cognitive processes, brain networks, mental processes, unconscious processes	Any problems require experts in those bad or difficult life situations and how they can be changed; and this will include others who have had life experiences in those same contexts
Any problems only require a single 'therapist' since the problem is internal	This will require a variety of people since no single person will have experience in so many possible life contexts
To fix problems you have to 'fix the person'	To support the person and help them you need to work with the person and a group of people to 'fix their life situations'
Therapy can be conducted in a neutral environment away from the person's contexts	Helping and supporting the person needs engagement with their life contexts to some degree
The therapy can be done just using language because you are trying to elicit their 'internal' problems and fix them	Just changing how a person talks can have some positive effects for them but if their situation is not changed it will not help in the long run and they will be reshaped
The therapy is independent of outside context, so the backgrounds and life contexts of both the person and the therapist are not really important, since you are trying to fix internal processes	The 'therapy' is fundamentally dependent upon the life histories and contexts of all those involved

A heads-up

My first task then will be to briefly go through some of the key terms used in therapy and psychology which *disguise* such external contexts and pretend that 'people do what they do' because of hidden and usually mysterious things occurring 'inside' people. Please note that I am not saying that the terms below are all wrong. The observations and experiences which prompt the use of these words, as I have hopefully made clear, are not in question at all, just our discourses about them. If we think in terms of the 'internal' person being affected, then we will try to 'fix the person' rather than trying to change their contexts (Figure 1.2). And 'internal' explanations also always open the door for blaming the victim when things do not change in therapy. So, these terms below are not wrong, they are everyday attempts to speak about what cannot easily be spoken, but they fail because they deceptively phrase them as something hidden inside a person and ignore the life contexts which have actually shaped them.

- *Psychology.* As I have argued above and elsewhere (Guerin, 2016a, 2020a), the whole enterprise of psychology has been an attempt to avoid analysing situations or contexts by instead talking about the causes of what people do as if these originate inside the person and are hidden from view. This shows, when you consider which phenomena are the ones we even label as 'psychological' in the first place; they are ones for which we cannot see an easy external context shaping the observable behaviours. The effects over time of living in bad life situations is a clear case where we do not see the bad situation as a clear 'object' and so we call any effects on the person 'psychological in origin', or something similar, "It must be something psychological". But this is tautological and not an explanation at all.
- *Internalized.* Another term which tries to talk about the observed changes in people's behaviour invokes the 'internal' directly. We say that the person has 'internalized' the issue or problem. This again is tautological, vague, and explains nothing; while again I am not denying that the observations that provoke the use of this term are real and not in dispute. As a cue for analysis, 'internalized' often really reflects that the issue is something about language and how the person is *talking about their own changes in behaviour.* So often one therapeutic clue will be to look for *discourse changes* in the person's behaviour when this term starts being used. They have not 'internalized', but they have markedly changed the ways they talk due to contexts in their social relationships (Chapter 7). A common situation where this term is used is when the person's talking is being punished by most of the people around them and so they stop saying things out loud.
- *Traumatic.* Once again, the later behaviours following bad life situations are frequently 'explained' by saying that the person was 'traumatized' or has

'held the trauma inside them'. Again, this does not explain anything and is tautological, even though the suffering observed or experienced is very real. 'Internal triggers' are also used to give some agency to the traumas being 'inside' us. One clue for analysis here is that when these terms are used the person has usually stopped a lot of their prior behaviours, especially talking out loud, and doing this has changed their life. The therapeutic clue is to look for those contexts which have punished or stopped their prior behaviours and do something about those.

- *Personality*. Changes from living in chronic bad life situations are often 'explained' by talking and thinking about the person as having 'a changed personality'. A person's 'personality' is just an abstract word for the common patterns they have been shaped to behave in their life situations: if you have a stable life context you will have stable ways of behaving shaped; if you have unstable external life situations you will (seem to) have an unstable personality (Fromene & Guerin, 2014). So, calling something a 'personality change' gives us a clue for analysis that the person now has a new stable or chronic bad life situation, which is continuing to shape their new 'personality'. The DSM, of course, is replete with such tautological 'explanations' under the guise of 'personality disorders'.

- *Brain changes*. As outlined elsewhere (Chapter 6), all changes of context and subsequent changes in behaviour involve the brain, but the brain itself is not *originating* these behaviour changes. So, while the brain is clearly involved, and correlations will always be found, it is not the source that needs changing when people are suffering. It is a convenient 'explanation' for anything a person does, however, especially with difficult-to-see external shaping contexts.

- *Emotional*. 'Emotional turmoil' and 'emotional issues' are also used as 'explanations' for someone having a bad life situation and later showing new behaviours. The 'emotion' is talked about as something 'inside' a person that vaguely stays there and then *these emotions drive* (originate) any new behaviours as if they were an agent. For a social contextual view (Guerin, 2020a), emotions are behaviours we do when (1) in bad or new situations, (2) we need to respond, but (3) we have no discourses or other behaviours for the audience requiring the response (more in Chapter 7). Such emotional responses are certainly prevalent in bad life situations; but, like the brain, they are not a 'causal' explanation for anything. So once again, the observations and experiences referred to by these words are very real, but the words cannot be used to explain anything.

- *Unconscious*. This is an earlier form of using hidden and metaphorical 'explanations' when the situations or contexts are not easily observed. Instead, it was said that the 'unconscious' has been affected and that the 'unconscious' is an agent that will later drive people to do things, so they will behave differently. The unconscious then turns out to be our external life worlds which are shaping what we do, say, and think, and a large part of this is our discourses (Lacan). Think of the 'unconscious' as all the life contexts in which you are embedded but which you cannot easily observe affecting you.

- *Deep and surface.* A common metaphor that functions in the same (wrong) way in everyday life, as well as professional writings, is the deep/surface metaphor. This is also an attribution strategy which does not really explain anything. "While the person seemed ok on the surface, deep inside things were brewing". Nice words, but metaphorical only. There is no 'deep inside the person' (except for their guts). As a clue for analysis and therapy, deep usually means 'more hidden' and usually refers to situations in which discourses which have been heavily punished (externally) are prevalent.

- *Meaning.* A very common last resort of explaining behaviour where contexts cannot easily be seen is to use 'meaning'. Typically, it is said that the person is doing what they are doing because they are 'searching for meaning', or 'need meaning in their life'. Once again, it is not disputed that there are important behaviours and experiences involved in such cases when this word is invoked, but rather that 'meaning' is an abstract word which does not explain at all. A better attempt is needed to say what this purported 'meaning' is doing in their concrete life (Chapter 6).

- *Information* and *processing.* I will finish with two words that have plagued and misguided more recent psychology and now everyday talk. Both these terms avoid looking for the external contexts which shape our uses of language, especially the social context, and instead refer to abstract and socially free 'internal' states, which appear to operate independently of the real social world. These two words imply that we are not influenced or shaped by our discursive communities to talk and think in certain way; rather, we *non-socially* 'take in' and 'process' non-social 'information'. These words sidestep the reality that our words and thoughts are shaped entirely by social contexts (Chapter 7) and can only pretend that we have a socially independent 'inside person' who deals with 'pure' information. As we will see, 'internal' metaphors are frequently resorted to when there are observations and experiences about our discourses or uses of language, but these always are shaped by social contexts and are not independently existing and non-social 'inside' the person. That has only arisen from the discursive strategy of using the words 'information' and 'processing' (you can see this starting in the 1950s psychology) and they miss the point of language use entirely and so explain nothing.

I will finish with one example of these word changes. In this case, people have correctly noticed that when there have been traumatic life events for a person that there will be important effects which cause suffering (the observations and experiences are not in doubt). But instead of looking for the contexts shaping these occurrences, the changes have lazily been labelled as the effects of 'internal personality changes', instead of observing all the 'external' contextual changes which have occurred for such a person.

This came from a recent anonymous meme and listed what the meme claimed "Unhealed trauma can look like":

- low sense of self worth
- codependency in relationships
- fear of being abandoned
- putting your needs aside for other people
- craving for external validation
- an innate feeling of shame
- not being able to tolerate conflict
- always fearing what might happen next
- resisting positive change
- tolerating abusive behaviours from others
- difficulty standing up for yourself and asserting boundaries
- being overly agreeable

Most of those items on the list cannot be observed and so they cannot 'look like' anything—they can only be reported as words and cannot be used as an explanation. But my key message is that the observations reported obviously have some basis in experience, but since nothing observable can be found, they are attributed to abstract words taking advantage of the consensus that they must reside 'inside' the person. However, by relegating the potentially observable life changes in a person's contexts to be hidden inside somewhere, we miss ways to support the person by changing the bad contexts to which they have been subjected. Spending time with longer and better observations of the 'external' life contexts shaping the suffering would be a more useful way to go. And that is precisely what this book is attempting to show you how do.

References

Bentley, A. F. (1941a/1975). The human skin: Philosophy's last line of defense. In A. F. Bentley, *Inquiry into inquiries: Essays in social theory*. Westport, Connecticut: Greenwood Press.

Bentley, A. F. (1941b). The behavioral superfice. *Psychological Review*, 48, 39–59.

Edwards, D. & Potter, J. (1993). Language and causation: A discursive action model of description and attribution. *Psychological Review*, 100, 23–41.

Fromene, R. & Guerin, B. (2014). Talking to Australian Indigenous clients with borderline personality disorder labels: Finding the context behind the diagnosis. *The Psychological Record*, 64, 569–579.

Guerin, B. (2016a). *How to rethink psychology: New metaphors for understanding people and their behavior*. London: Routledge.

Guerin, B. (2016b). *How to rethink human behavior: A practical guide to social contextual analysis*. London: Routledge.

Guerin, B. (2017). *How to rethink mental illness: The human contexts behind the labels*. London: Routledge.

Guerin, B. (2020a). *Turning psychology into social contextual analysis.* London: Routledge.
Guerin, B. (2020b). *Turning psychology into a social science.* London: Routledge.
Guerin, B. (2020c). *Turning mental health into social action.* London: Routledge.
Hinton, D. (2016). *Existence: A story.* Boulder: Shambhala.

2 What are the contexts for therapies you need to be aware of?

There are a *lot* of 'schools' of therapy, most claiming to be different and usually better, and this is unlike most of science (Percy, 1985). Some are based on different talking, thinking or theories, while others are based on different techniques or methods (Benson & van Loon, 2012; Corsini & Wedding, 2010; Frank, 1975; Halbur & Halbur, 2006; McLeod, 2010; Osipow, Walsh & Tosi, 1984; Sharf, 2016).

In the next four chapters, I will start to 'dissect' the whole idea and practice of therapy. This is dissection not demolition. Unlike some other attempts at this (Masson, 1994), I am not going to conclude that therapy is a waste of time. I will conclude that:

- we are still not sure what is helping those people who say that they benefit from therapy (without doubting that it does sometimes help)
- the talk or discourses that are given for what happens in therapy are most commonly *fictions* (whether medical models, psychological models or alternative therapies)
- the real issues of 'mental health' are only indirectly being addressed by the way current forms of therapy are conducted
- probably a lot of the 'successes' of therapy are due to situational changes occurring over time anyway, or due to not following up those people who withdraw from therapy
- we can do a lot better by exploring new practices, observing the person and their life contexts, and discarding most of the discourses around therapy which are restricting us

In this chapter I will first look simply at what therapy is, and then examine all the contexts for therapy being done at all, including social, economic, and political contexts (Marks, 2017). I will then explore all the behaviours occurring in therapy in the following three chapters:

- the discourses or language use around therapy, *what therapists say they do?*
- what 'treatment' methods do therapists use, *what therapists do, in general?*

DOI: 10.4324/9781003300571-3

- how do therapists behave with their clients, what are different *components* of this singular word 'therapy', and *how therapists respond more specifically in therapy with another human being?*

Some of this will be done by a close exegesis of 19 common psychotherapies. My approach to doing this is based on my experience of working as follows:

- observe therapists and take what you *see* seriously
- listen to them talk about *what they actually do* and take this seriously except when they stray from concrete descriptions and use any type of abstract language
- ignore how they explain what they do, why they do it, or how they market it
- do not let the second two points put you off taking the first point seriously
- all 'therapies' have multiple component events occurring, any one of which could be what is causing the change and not what the therapist is saying causes any changes which might occur

We need to remember that what therapists do *can* be useful and beneficial even if their theories and discourses are whacky—and I include the medical models and the DSM here as whacky as well (Davies, 2014; Guerin, 2017; Johnstone & Boyle, 2018; Watson, 2019). So, do not let whacky and abstract theorizing convince you that what a therapist does is not useful; and do not let a perfectly sensible and consistent theory which makes a very moving story convince you that what the therapist does is useful either.

What is therapy, anyway? Situating therapy in its contexts

To start, I looked on the *www* for 'therapy' and got the sorts of answers shown in Box 2.1. You can try likewise.

Box 2.1 Descriptions of therapy from various websites

Treatment intended to relieve or heal a disorder: 'A course of antibiotic therapy'; The treatment of mental or psychological disorders by psychological means: 'He is currently in therapy'

Therapy helps people talk about their feelings. It helps them work through problems and learn new skills. When they do this, they start to communicate better and do better. People need therapy for different reasons.

There are five major stages that we will look at today. Here is what they are: Stage 1 – Initial Disclosure, Stage 2 – In depth Exploration, Stage 3 – Commitment to action, Stage 4 – Counseling intervention, and Stage 5 – Evaluation, Termination or Referral. Let's look at what each of those mean.

Therapy can be an effective treatment for a host of mental and emotional problems. Simply talking about your thoughts and feelings with a supportive person can often make you feel better. It can be very healing, in and of itself, to voice your worries or talk about something that's weighing on your mind.

A therapist is a licensed medical professional that evaluates, diagnoses, and treats people with emotional and mental disorders. In treating diagnosed mental disorders and nervous disorders or other emotional issues, they apply family systems theories and psychotherapeutic techniques.

Therapy, also called psychotherapy or counseling, is the process of meeting with a therapist to resolve problematic behaviors, beliefs, feelings, relationship issues, and/or somatic responses (sensations in the body).

Therapy is the process of meeting with a counsellor or psychotherapist for the purpose of resolving problematic behaviours, beliefs, feelings and related physical symptoms. Therapy uses an interpersonal relationship to help develop the client's self-understanding and to make changes in his or her life.

In psychotherapy, psychologists help people of all ages live happier, healthier and more productive lives. Psychologists apply research-based techniques to help people develop more effective habits. There are several approaches to psychotherapy, including cognitive-behavioral, interpersonal and psychodynamic, among others, that help people work through their problems. Psychotherapy is a collaborative treatment based on the relationship between an individual and a psychologist. A psychologist provides a supportive environment that allows you to talk openly with someone who is objective, neutral and nonjudgmental. Most therapy focuses on individuals, although psychotherapists also work with couples, families and groups.

With a little variation, they are all saying very similar things:

- therapy is when someone with some sorts of problems in life talks to another person
- they are not just ordinary problems but special problems (although what these are is left abstract)
- the life problems are something 'internal' to the person, or something 'psychological' (Chapter 1)
- with a therapist they try and solve the problems
- there is only one therapist
- sometimes just talking about the problems can be beneficial
- these problems are commonly named as beliefs, mental events, perceptions, feelings, emotions, or thoughts
- some say explicitly that these problems are due to a 'disorder'
- therapists also aim to change 'problematic' behaviours and social relationship problems

- some try to teach useful skills; most try to solve specific problems just by talking
- others help just to 'work through their problems' (whatever this means)
- they all involve meeting and talking with a stranger they do not know ("who is objective, neutral and nonjudgmental")
- there is also a hidden assumption that you must pay money for this other person to talk; it is a contractual arrangement

It is worthwhile reading these descriptions over, finding more yourself online, and discussing with others. See what you can add to my list above of the broadly assumed *contexts* for therapy. We will come back to these and a lot more, but these are your first candidates for the contexts of doing modern therapy. And there are major problems with all of them! ("Simply talking about your thoughts and feelings with a supportive person *can often* make you feel better").

A common theme during these next few chapters is that all therapies are actually doing very similar things, probably with similar outcomes, but using all sorts of different words to describe what they think is going on. After that we will discover that 'doing therapy' hides a lot of *component events* which are not mentioned, and which might really be the basis of any help that succeeds. But all the above descriptions of therapy are very abstract and general.

Filling in more of the broad social, historical, economic, and political contexts of modern mainstream therapies

Let me first put more of a historical context onto therapy. There was not always therapy. It appeared in the late 1800s, and only really became as we know it now from about the 1950s. As described elsewhere (Guerin, 2020a, Chapter 1; Rose, 1999), there were particular social and political contexts for this. It did not emerge 'naturally' from 'pastoral' care. It arose because the nature of our social relationships in society changed drastically, because family groups and communities could no longer solve all of people's problems and conflicts, and because of the huge societal and political changes in the way of life people were forced to live.

Modern mainstream forms of therapy are now thoroughly embedded in our modern way of life (Guerin, 2020a, Chapter 1). This includes the capitalist economy, the neoliberal administrative bureaucracies to govern and order populations, government rules and policies governing who can obtain therapy with government support (since it is too costly for most people to pay themselves), and the government-ordained hierarchies of power within these various societal systems, especially the medical system.

Ever since governments gave power to medical personnel to judge and assist with 'mental health' problems (Guerin, 2020a, Chapter 1; Miller & Rose, 1994), psychiatrists have been the most powerful of the therapeutic specialists. They and clinical psychologists are about the only ones who can legally judge 'what is wrong' with a person *in the absence of other evidence*, and they can even go against the words of the person themself. And the category system invented by psychiatrists has dominion over defining 'what is wrong', despite its non-scientific foundations (APA, 2013; Caplan, 1995; Davies, 2014).

The neoliberal approach to mainstream therapy is seen in its thinking, rationale, and funding: there is a problem; we consult experts; they assess and categorize the problem; they recommend a 'standard' procedure for solving the problem 'discovered' by the category of problem; they then use the associated procedures to solve the problem; and, hey presto, a cure! And in good neoliberal fashion, this must all be done in the most efficient and quick way.

This works mostly fine with truly medical problems. I have an eye problem, I consult an expert, they test and categorize a specific medical condition, and there is already a standard treatment associated for each medical condition (albeit not always effective in every case).

Unfortunately, *almost every piece of this chain fails with 'mental health'*. It is now very unclear who really is an expert in matters of 'mental health'. Psychiatrists, and later, clinical psychologists, were given this power *by governments* dating back to the late 1800s, when new symptoms appeared which had no easy explanations; and so the problems were handed to medical experts who eventually morphed into psychiatrists (Guerin, 2020a, Chapter 1; Miller & Rose, 1994), despite finding no evidence of a medical basis to what are called 'mental health' issues. Psychologists have also developed models of what happens to a person when they exhibit 'mental health' problems, but these have been widely criticized and are abstract and not linked to everyday life and contexts.

The 'experts' have meanwhile developed a category system (DSM) for the 'mental health' problem which mimics the medical versions, but is seriously flawed (Bentall, 2006; Davies, 2014; Guerin, 2020a; Johnstone, 2014; Johnstone & Boyle, 2018; Kinderman, 2019; Rose, 1999; Watson, 2019). And moreover, *there are no treatments associated with the categories anyway,* in the way that all other medical diagnoses have. So 'mental health' treatments are made to *resemble* medical models and *resemble* neoliberal efficiency in procuring cures, but these are total fictions. Meanwhile, rates of 'mental health' problems continue to increase and people suffer, and it is blamed on brain problems.

These social, societal, economic, and cultural contexts of modernity also feature in the concrete settings of most mainstream therapies. Here are some of those therapy contexts touched on so far to consider, and to analyze the impact on any outcomes (Guerin, 2016):

- conducted in an office away from the person's life contexts
- the person pays money for the therapy, so any mutual obligations between the two persons rest on a contract rather than more personal ties, and the contractual obligations and any responsibilities cease after the contract ends
- there is a single therapist
- talking is almost exclusively the only vehicle for change
- usually meet for 50-minute sessions once a week or less

- conducted with a stranger (who therefore does not know the person's contexts at all, has no obligation to the person beyond the monetary and professional contract, and is not connected in any way to the person's family or social networks; Guerin, 2016)
- this stranger has little or no experience of the person's bad life situations (no participation with the person and probably little personal life experience in such contexts)
- the therapists usually have little or no experience themselves of living in many of life's worst conditions, and less of any intersectional effects
- there are usually large social and economic power differentials between the therapist and the 'client'

This is not a good prognosis for a 'cure'!

Societal contexts of therapy: details of the "therapy bubble"

Figures 2.1 to 2.7 put some of these ideas into graphic form to help you visualize the contexts and see more than I have written about here. Most importantly, whether therapist or recipient, picture yourself in similar therapy situations and not only analyse new contexts I have missed, but also notice what is different from your own experience to my figures and analyze the further contexts in your own case which make this different. For example, your therapist might meet you outside an office sometimes, *but* what makes this possible since it goes against 'professional conduct'? As a therapist, you might not charge the full fee to some clients who are economically struggling, but what are the extra contexts that allow this happen in the first place (and do not attribute this to some wonderful 'inner' personality of your own).

What I really want to make clear in all this is that the therapeutic situation, which I will call the "*therapy bubble*", is *not* context free. Therapy is sometimes presented as a context which is free of constraints, where the recipient is free to say whatever they like, and the therapist can be open and honest. Remember one of the definitions given earlier of the therapist "who is objective, neutral and nonjudgmental". This is an illusion as we will see, based on the western illusion that we are all free, independent 'individuals' who can choose to do and say whatever we want. Rather, the therapeutic situation is *loaded* with social, societal, governmental, and bureaucratic constraints on both parties. And as I explained in Chapter 1, we can only imagine this situation as context-free because of our 'internal' models of human behaviour.

Figure 2.1 shows the basic therapy situation when conducted in person. Nothing much really changes for online therapy, except for a few new ways of responding to each other when not physically present.

In the office there are two people talking. The one on the right is the therapist and the one on the left the 'client', 'patient', or 'consumer', depending upon the framework of the therapist (McLaughlin, 2009). I will use

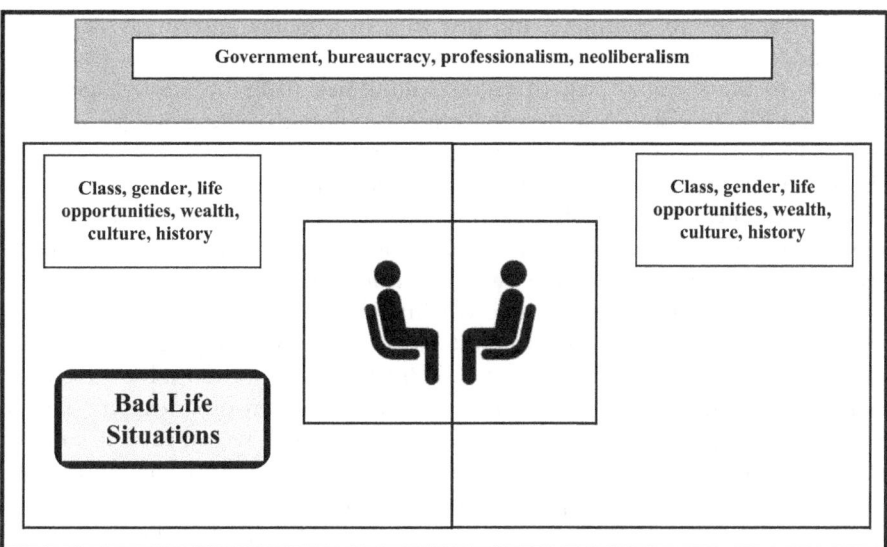

Figure 2.1 The basic contexts for therapy

'recipient' although sometimes the pair are talked about as 'collaborating', even though this is usually a very one-sided collaboration. They are nowadays almost always seated and facing, although other positions have been used in the past.

In the bottom left-hand corner, *outside the office*, are the bad life situations in which the recipient is embedded (Chapter 8). While physically outside the office, these bad life situations are in many ways truly present within the office as well. Much of the recipient's actions, talking, thinking, and emotions have been shaped by these bad life situations. This outside shaping does not get removed simply by 50 minutes of shaping from the therapist within the bubble, except as a transient distraction.

Each of the two persons has also been shaped by their more specific groups, families, and acquaintances, and the opportunities which have been available in their lives. This can be talked about as class, opportunism, wealth, culture, etc. This main point is that these are likely to be very different for each of the two people.

In a similar way, illustrated at the top, this whole therapy situation is shaped by contexts arranged by governments, bureaucracies, professional associations, and law courts. There are ways in which the therapist is *supposed* to behave and talk, and ways they are *not allowed* to behave and talk. Whether they wish to or not. As mentioned earlier, I have talked with therapists who go walking with their clients instead of sitting in an office, but they almost all have to keep this quiet from their colleagues and administrators.

Inside the therapy bubble the therapist at least is constrained (shaped) to behave in certain professional ways, and the conversation and conduct should be reasonable and normal. There is the neoliberal context imposed that there is work to do, a job to complete, and this must be efficient and timely. There is also a hidden context of economic exchange, that the recipient must pay contractually to the therapist, whether this is done personally or through government subsidies. In either case this will imply a number of life consequences for the recipient, making therapy unavailable to many (Goodman, Pugach, Skolnik, & Smith, 2013; Santiago, Kaltman, & Miranda, 2013).

Another context which is often ignored but will become important (Figure 2.7 below; Chapter 7) is the discursive context within the therapy bubble, and how this derives from the two people's own historical contexts.

A final point to make is that overwhelmingly, *there is a single therapist*. This derives, I believe, from what was said in Chapter 1. If 'psychological' problems are in the 'mind' or ''mental processes' of an individual, then we can solve these by a single 'mind' expert and we do not have to worry about any other experts. This is unlike, for example, having a serious leg injury where you would have all sorts of professionals working with you on different aspects of the problems: surgeons, doctors, physiotherapists, occupational therapists, home carers, etc. The reason for pointing this out is that – with the framework I will develop later in this book – the 'mental health' problems are not 'in your head' but in your life world; so it makes total sense to involve a lot more people, since you are not just dealing with a fictitious 'mind' problem but need to be supported and assisted in many aspects of your life worlds, which require different expertise.

Figure 2.2 emphasizes that the recipient of therapy is living most of the time in bad life situations and being shaped accordingly (Chapter 7). The therapy

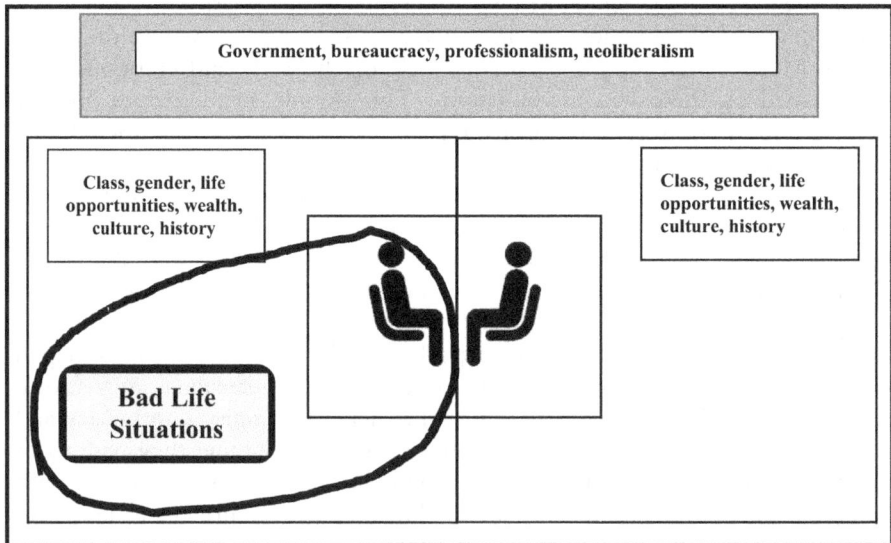

Figure 2.2 The key contexts for the recipients of therapy are bad life situations they are struggling with, but these are kept remote from the office setting

office, however, is a very different and remote environment and might make it difficult to respond in the same way, and the behaviours, talking, and thoughts in their 'outside' life can look peculiar when viewed within the office and taken 'out of context'. This is even more so if the therapist has not experienced those situations firsthand.

> *And those who were seen dancing were thought to be insane by those who could not hear the music.*
>
> (Variously attributed to Nietzsche, Anne Louise Germaine de Staël, anonymous, and many others)

This also means that for the therapist to take the bad life situations seriously, *the recipient can only convey this by talking.* There are several problems arising from this, not least of which is that the recipient might not be able to accurately convey in words their bad situations, even if the therapist were to take them seriously. Further, many of these bad life situations *cannot* be put into words easily.

Figure 2.3 shows that the therapy context forms a little hub around the two people, even if their major behaviours are being shaped elsewhere. This "therapy bubble" context has several effects worth noting. This isolated and repetitive bubble shapes up its own 'cultural behaviours' (Guerin, 2016) in several ways.

First, the 'bubble' will build up idiosyncrasies within the therapy situation not known to others, especially if it continues over some time and remains isolated from other people (due to government and professional rules about confidentiality, of course). There will be patterns created unintentionally, which might be similar across a lot of recipients of the one therapist, but also purely specific to individual recipients. The therapy bubble is in fact what I describe as a cultural behaviour (Guerin, 2016).

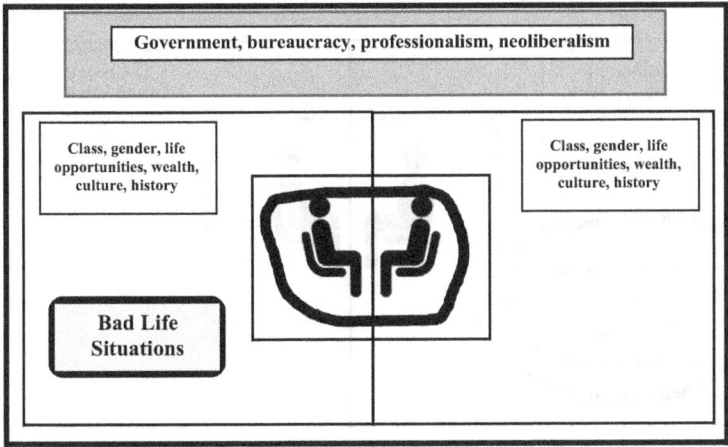

Figure 2.3 The "therapy bubble" resulting from trying to remove contexts

Second, the world itself does not enter the therapy bubble *while it is happening*. The talk continues uninterrupted and is confidential within the bubble. This can have both good and bad effects, of course, which you should analyze more carefully. But what goes on is not monitored by others usually, and in fact legally it is meant to be confidential and protected. These are, as is well known, typical conditions for building cult behaviours and beliefs in which both parties agree but no one else does, and there are no consequences because of the confidentiality.

Third, this also means that language is the major behaviour occurring in therapy and there are perils with relying on language (Guerin, 2020b, Chapter 7). As mentioned earlier, *if the recipient is not able to articulate their bad life situations* then the therapist is likely to draw wrong conclusions and make inaccurate explanations. Further, the reliance on language alone means that both people can easily lie to the other, persuade them, or pretend to be trustworthy. These strategies are easy to develop and maintain when there is no outside monitoring and when only words are being used and no other actions observed.

Fourth, any language changes which are taught or else unknowingly shaped by the therapist are shaped within the therapy bubble and there is no guarantee that these will function when the person is back in their world. The new discourses shaped within therapy (new statements, new beliefs, new rhetorical strategies, new rejoinders, marketing statements, strategies to stop certain thoughts or talking, etc.), can easily be punished, reshaped, sidelined, gaslighted, or overpowered when the person gets back into their usual world (Figure 2.4).

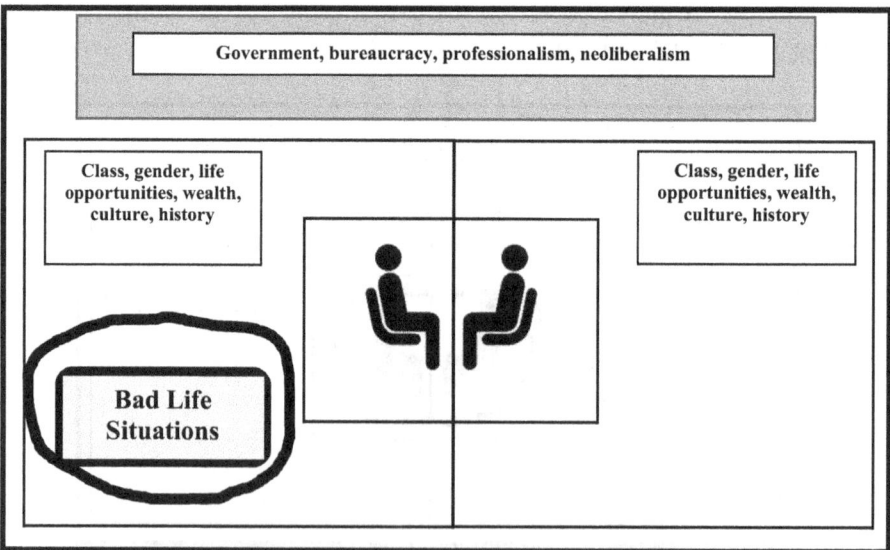

Figure 2.4 The person's real problems, their bad life situations, remain outside of the therapy except for what the person is able to talk about

Finally, while skills other than language can be taught within the therapy bubble, most skills taught now are language skills (labelled as 'cognitive'). The problems with teaching language, mentioned above, apply equally to teaching 'behavioural skills'.

Figure 2.4 emphasizes some points already made. There are negative effects of the recipient's bad life situations which are not observable, talkable, or engageable within therapy bubbles. In physical medicine this is like a person having bad allergies but meeting in a doctor's office so that both can only *guess* what might be causing the allergy. Or when the 'symptoms' of the medical complaint do not occur inside the doctor's office (like a reverse white coat hypertension). Diagnosis and treatment are then completely reliant on how well both the doctor and patient can *remember* possible allergy-inducing objects or events, and whether these can even be articulated and observed in any case. Common allergy-inducing objects or events can be guessed (without real certainly) by highly experienced doctors, but it is very much guesswork until allergy experts are sent to the person's house to investigate directly.

In our present case of therapy, things are much worse than this. It has been unclear for 150 years what exactly in a person's life is shaping their 'presenting' behaviours (unlike allergies), so it is even more reliant on guesswork, even for experienced therapists (Chapter 1). Hence the 150 years of writing and rewriting fictions about the 'causes' of 'mental health' problems.

Figure 2.5 explains a lot of the context for therapy. Many of those critics blaming therapists for not doing X are not aware of the governmental contexts which might prevent them from doing X. There are all sorts of societal and

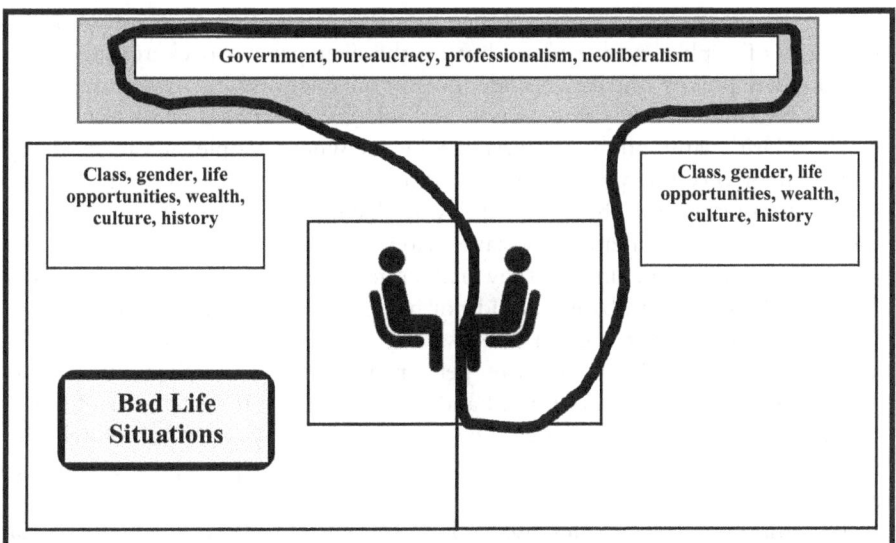

Figure 2.5 Some societal contexts limiting the behaviours possible in a therapy bubble

professional rules and regulations which can be punished if not followed. In general, these are meant to protect people, but, being verbal rules, they cannot encompass life properly (Guerin, 2020b, Chapter 7) and can make things worse. Many questions of "But why don't you do X in therapy" are answered here (but without really solving anything).

There are two more serious concerns here. Both these concerns are being addressed by 'consumer' help, support and legal assistance, which makes it clear that the problems are real. The real thing to note is that I am not talking about the (hopefully) rare cases of therapists directly abusing their power imbalance; but rather, the ever-present differences lying in the contextual background and how that *inadvertently* shapes what goes on in the therapy bubble all the time.

First, in almost all therapy contexts with psychiatrists and doctors, and in many contexts with clinical psychologists, society has given strong legal and bureaucratic powers *to the therapist*. These often remain just a threat in the contextual background but can be enforced if necessary. Psychiatrists have been given the rights to have a person incarcerated through a historical quirk (Guerin, 2020a, Chapter 1). The problem is not a few rogue psychiatrists who might abuse this power, which can be tempting when they do not know what else to do, but the ever-present power differential lying in the background, which can shape all the behaviours and thoughts of the recipient without anything being overtly mentioned. People are not stupid, and they know who can do what to whom inside the therapy bubble.

The second big concern is that this unequal power means that the therapist always has a way of being correct in both facts and judgements, with little chance of redress for recipients. Once again, this is not to focus on perhaps a few cases of explicit power abuse but on the ever-present background context this implicit power imbalance engenders in all relationships. Expertise will be seen as unequal whether true or not, and whether overtly used or not.

There are many other potential problems when people are in a therapy bubble with very unequal power according to those outside the bubble. Once out of the bubble, the therapist will always have professional others to support the beliefs and judgements they have made. The recipients will often have no one to support them, since if they had someone they could talk to and solve their problems they probably would not have gone to therapy in the first place. That is, the discourses learned and used by therapists come from professional and governmental classes and can get strong backing whether true or not. Psychiatric theories about the mind and drugs are just some examples of this. In this arena of therapy, the phrase "The customer is always right" absolutely does *not* hold. Hence the strong need for 'consumer' help, support, and legal assistance.

The imposed societal rules also include the current western values of neoliberalism, which focuses upon stable nuclear family relationships and employment as the goals for everyone, with a strong commitment to the (dubious) benefits of being competitive in society. Once again, therapists will not be

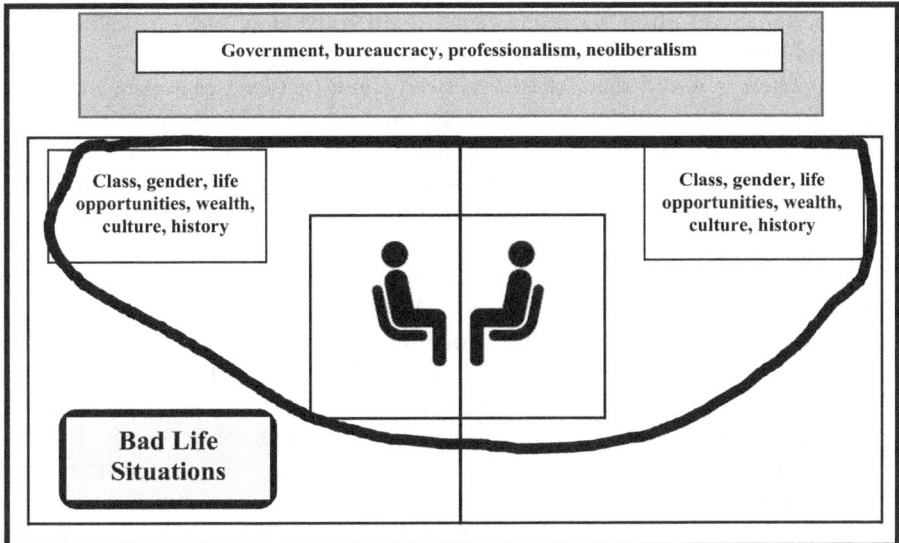

Figure 2.6 Differing life contexts between recipients and therapists

overtly preaching neoliberal values, that is not what I mean, but because of the constraints which therapists are under, such values will be part of the goals of therapy. Neoliberal views also promulgate that we are individuals who can control and choose what we say and do and therefore can be held responsible. Many recipients write, from firsthand experience, that blaming them for their behaviours happens, either overtly or covertly, inside the therapy bubble.

Figure 2.6 is meant to evoke the differing contexts in the life backgrounds of therapist and recipient. Once upon a time, when the theory was that 'mental disorders' were universal across a large number of people and related to 'internal' or brain problems (Chapter 1), the actual background context of a therapist, and any differences to their recipients, was not a big issue. The therapists were experts in these decontextualized 'internal' problems, which needed (supposedly) universal knowledge and treatments so the backgrounds were not important. However, with 'universal' mental health or 'psychological' problems being debunked as the locus of the problems (Chapter 1), the background contexts of the people in the bubble becomes extremely relevant (Chapter 8).

Of special importance is the therapist's lack of real experience (rather than verbal knowledge) of the bad life situations. But just experiencing bad life situations is not enough to help, since in that case the recipient could do without the therapist, but what is needed is the *experiential knowledge* of what occurs in bad life situations, what strategies evolve in them, and how to change the bad situations. Without any 'street' knowledge of these, the therapist will be limited in what they can do and will be shaped to just make the recipient feel better in the short term and teach them some new ways of talking—but the bad situations will still remain.

So, when it is said that "therapists need some firsthand experience of living in these bad life situations", this needs more careful exploration. It is not a simple switch, such that *any* experience will be helpful, nor that no direct experience automatically means that the therapist is useless. Rather, it is experiencing and/or knowing all the intricacies of being shaped in bad life situations, and the complexities of outcomes, that is important.

Figure 2.7 is similar to Figure 2.6 but with one big difference—it specifically focuses on the different *language uses* and *discourses* between therapist and recipient. We get most things done in our lives now through using language, so this is of special concern. Both the societal inequalities (Figure 2.7) and the background contexts of the two people in the bubble mean that the therapist is most likely to be the more persuasive within the relationship (Frank, 1975). It also means that there can be miscommunications because of backgrounds if this is a big difference.

This is another positive aspect of therapists having some experience with bad life situations, that they also know what can be put into words and what cannot, and they will know some of the idiomatic ways in which language is used. An example I heard recently was of a person being released from an emergency ward saying that he "felt like a rock star", a common expression meaning to feel happy. This was overheard by the medical staff and taken to be a delusion, at which point he was readmitted!

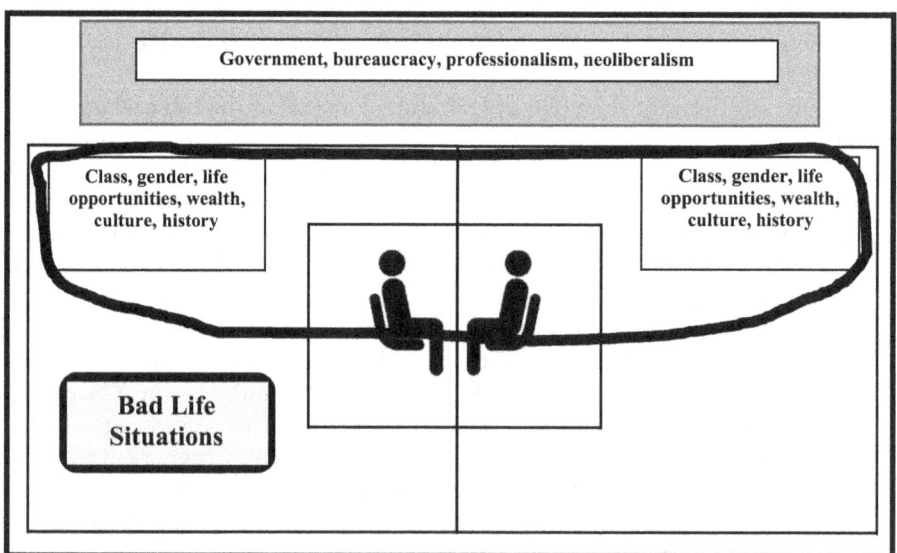

Figure 2.7 Differing discursive life contexts between recipients and therapists

Of course, the therapists all have their own idiomatic uses of language (Chapter 3), which range from 'scientific' jargon to new age explanations for problems, but with the power imbalance described earlier, these need to be taken seriously by the recipients, at least when inside the bubble—rather than the reverse. Currently recipients need to listen and understand the therapist's theories, jargon, and marketing, but not the reverse.

As will become clear with contextual views of language use and thinking (Chapter 7), language use and discourse are not primarily about the words and phrases used. Discourse means how language is used to manage our social behaviours and get people to do things, and therefore about all the power and reciprocities in people's lives. Given this real context for language use, we have seen (Figures 2.5 and 2.6), the ability to accomplish things with words will be vastly different between therapists and recipients of therapy.

Finally, in Chapters 7 and 8 we will discover that many of the 'mental health' behaviours involve the person's language use failing to have any effects. This is not due to poor language skills or miscommunications, but due to their outside audiences and social relationships no longer supporting their talk as social behaviour. This means that how a therapist responds becomes contentious since they are likely to be facing someone with a lifetime of their language being useless to accomplish anything, and only ever getting responses of punishment, neglect, or defiant opposition. I will address this further in Chapter 5 (Guerin, Ball, & Ritchie, 2021).

References

American Psychiatric Association (2013). *The diagnostic and statistical manual of mental disorders* (5th Ed.). Washington: APA.

Benson, N. & van Loon, B. (2012). *Psychotherapy: A graphic guide*. London: Icon Books.

Bentall, R. P. (2006). Madness explained: Why we must reject the Kraepelinian paradigm and replace it with a 'complaint-orientated' approach to understanding mental illness. *Medical Hypotheses*, 66, 220–233.

Caplan, P. J. (1995). *They say you're crazy: How the world's most powerful psychiatrists decide who's normal*. NY: Life Long.

Corsini, R. J. & Wedding, D. (2010). *Current psychotherapies* (9th Ed.). NY: Brooks/Cole.

Davies, J. (2014). *Cracked: Why psychiatry is doing more harm than good*. London: Icon Books.

Frank, J. D. (1975). *Persuasion and healing: A comparative study of psychotherapy*. NY: Schocken Books.

Goodman, L. A., Pugach, M., Skolnik, A., & Smith, L. (2013). Poverty and mental health practice: Within and beyond the 50-minute hour. *Journal of Clinical Psychology: In Session*, 69, 182–190.

Guerin, B. (2016). *How to rethink human behavior: A practical guide to social contextual analysis*. London: Routledge.

Guerin, B. (2017). *How to rethink mental illness: The human contexts behind the labels*. London: Routledge.

Guerin, B. (2020a). *Turning mental health into social action.* London: Routledge.

Guerin, B. (2020b). *Turning psychology into social contextual analysis.* London: Routledge.

Guerin, B., Ball, M., & Ritchie, R. (2021). *Therapy in the absence of psychopathology and neoliberalism.* University of South Australia: Unpublished paper.

Halbur, D. A. & Halbur, K. V. (2006). *Developing your theoretical orientation in counselling and psychotherapy.* London: Pearson.

Johnstone, L. (2014). *A straight talking introduction to psychiatric diagnosis.* London: PCCS Books.

Johnstone, L., Boyle, M., Cromby, J., Dillon, J., Harper, D., Kinderman, P., ... Read, J. (2018). *The Power Threat Meaning Framework: Towards the identification of patterns in emotional distress, unusual experiences and troubled or troubling behaviour, as an alternative to functional psychiatric diagnosis.* Leicester, UK: British Psychological Society.

Kinderman, P. (2019). *A manifesto for mental health: Why we need a revolution in mental health care.* London: Palgrave Macmillan.

Marks, S. (2017). Psychotherapy in historical perspective. *History of the Human Sciences, 30,* 3–16.

Masson, J. M. (1994). *Against therapy.* Monroe, MN: Common Courage Press.

McLaughlin, H. (2009). What's in a name: 'Client', 'patient', 'customer', 'consumer', 'service user'—what's next? *British Journal of Social Work, 39,* 1101–1117.

McLeod, J. (2010). *The counsellor's workbook: Developing a personal approach.* London: Open University Press.

Miller, P. & Rose, N. (1994). On therapeutic authority: Psychoanalytical expertise under advanced liberalism. *History of the Human Sciences, 7,* 29–64.

Osipow, S. H., Walsh, W. B., & Tosi, D. J. (1984). *A survey of counselling methods.* IL: The Dorsey Press.

Percy, W. (1985). *Lost in the cosmos: The last self-help book.* NY: Picador.

Rose, N. (1999). *Governing the soul: The shaping of the private self* (2nd Ed.). London: Free Association Book.

Santiago, C. D., Kaltman, S., & Miranda, J. (2013). Poverty and mental health: How do low-income adults and children fare in psychotherapy? *Journal of Clinical Psychology: In Session, 69,* 115–126.

Sharf, R. S. (2016). *Theories of psychotherapy and counseling: Concepts and cases* (6th Ed.). Boston, MA: Cengage Learning.

Watson, J. (2019). *Drop the disorder: Challenging the culture of psychiatric diagnosis.* London: PCCS Books.

3   What do therapists say about what they do?

Theories and marketing of therapy

People are very poor at trying to explain behaviour, whether their own or that of other people (Chapter 1). They tend to be simplistic, and 'mono-causal', and only look at the salient parts of the environment to explain why people do what they do. And most everyday 'explanations' are not really explanations at all. This applies to explaining the inanimate world as well as human and animal behaviour. Just think of how you 'explain' the behaviours of your pets.

But there is one worse problem when it comes to explaining human behaviour. Most of what shapes people to do what they do is *not* immediately salient and is often not even present in the immediately vicinity (Guerin, 2016a, 2016b). What everyday people, as well as psychologists, do in these cases is to invent 'internal' fictions which *appear* to explain, and which, because they cannot be observed, cannot be easily disputed. Critically, the whole of psychology since its inception has been founded upon this discursive strategy of explanation: explaining what you cannot easily see by mind, spirit, brain processes, mental processes, cognitive processes, etc. (Chapter 1).

Another discursive phenomenon you need to be attuned to and observe is that when people do not know how to explain something, but are under pressure to do so, there are numerous ways to 'hedge' or 'mitigate' any responsibly or fault if what you say ends up being wrong and you mess up. I have already mentioned one of these hedges above, the use of *mentalisms* to hedge responsibility. If you explain a behaviour by some thing or 'process' inside the head or 'mind', or describe it as a 'mental' phenomenon, you are in fact hedging and not explaining anything. It is not observable so you can talk your way out of it easily.

Another common way of hedging responsibility is to begin using *abstract, general* or *ambiguous* language. It is more difficult for people to challenge abstract explanations since there are no concrete observations anyway; it is more difficult for people to challenge general or ambiguous explanations since no one knows what is meant really and the speaker can squirm out of responsibility. If you watch someone who is being challenged when they are trying to explain something, they will usually switch to using more abstract terms. Try this: ask someone you know to explain 'how cows make milk' and watch out for the

DOI: 10.4324/9781003300571-4

abstract words appearing (unless the person is an animal physiologist or biochemist).

Now the reason I mentioned these ways of hedging (there are many more, such as embedding the explanation into a longer story), is that they have supported the very foundations of psychology as a discipline for 150 years (Guerin, 2020a). Psychology has been built upon these two mistakes when trying to explain. When you do not know what is going on (which is most of the time for humans, unless you spend a lot of time observing them in their contexts), your explanations get accepted and protected by (1) making the causes hidden or unobservable, (2) making the causes very abstract, and (3) embedding your 'explanation' into a larger fictitious story. The first can be done by appealing to spirits and gods controlling human behaviour, but the 150 years of psychology as a separate discipline have been justified by allowing other unseeable realms called 'mental', 'mind', 'self', and 'psychological' to 'explain' instead. When questioned more and challenged, psychological theories go abstract and ambiguous very quickly, or 'authority' is used to shut down the conversation.

Another of the problems which leads us all to poor explanations of human behaviour is that the reasons we usually provide people for our own behaviour often consists simply of what we are 'thinking' when we do those behaviours, even though this thinking is not causing those behaviours to happen (Chapter 7; Guerin, 2020a). Instead, the 'thinking' is there to explain to other people, perhaps later, what we are doing and why (Guerin, 2020a), to justify, or to exaggerate. So, it often appears like what we say and think 'cause' what we do, but this is a confusion over two very different sorts of behaviours—the doing and the talking/thinking. Both are important, but they are for different parts of our lives, and one cannot be explained by the other. So, when asked why we are doing something we often just report what thoughts we had, even though these are not controlling or bringing about those behaviours.

There is more in discourse analysis which can help us weed out the talking by therapists from what they do, including a range of what I have called the '*perils of using language*' (Guerin, 2020a). But I will not go through these systematically and apply them to therapy here. Instead, I will just give an example from a classic and good book about psychotherapies. Look for the use of 'mentalisms' and abstractions:

> Psychotherapy tries to relieve a person's distress and improve his [sic] functioning by helping him to correct errors and resolve conflicts in his attitudes about himself and others. These attitudes are organized into systems existing at varying levels of consciousness and in harmonious or conflicting relationships with one another. They affect and are affected by emotional states, and changes in them are regularly accompanied by emotions. Healthy attitude systems are characterized by internal consistency and close correspondence with actual conditions. They thus lead to reliable, satisfactory social interactions, accompanied by a sense of competence, inner security, and well-being, which enables the person to modify

them readily when necessary. Unhealthy attitude systems are internally full of conflict and do not accurately correspond to circumstances, leading to experiences of frustration, failure, and alienation. Efforts to cope with or evade these feelings tend to be both self-perpetuating and self-defeating, resulting in cumulative, adaptational difficulties.

(Frank, 1975, pp. 44–45).

This is not radical psychology nor an extreme form of psychology, it is quite characteristic over the last 100 years for talking about therapy and human behaviour. Later in this chapter I will examine the goals for 19 different psychotherapies, and we will find little difference between them once the ambiguous and jargon (marketing) words are removed. But let us examine this passage more closely. Here are the abstract and mentalistic words which cannot be observed and are purely based in talking or theory (italics):

Psychotherapy *tries* to *relieve* a person's *distress* and improve his [sic] *functioning* by helping him to correct *errors* and *resolve* conflicts in his *attitudes* about himself and others. These *attitudes* are organized into *systems existing* at varying *levels* of *consciousness* and in harmonious or conflicting *relationships* with one another. They *affect* and are affected by *emotional states*, and changes in them are regularly accompanied by *emotions*. *Healthy attitude systems* are characterized by *internal consistency* and close *correspondence* with *actual* conditions. They thus *lead* to *reliable, satisfactory* social interactions, *accompanied* by a *sense* of *competence, inner security*, and *well-being*, which enables the person to *modify them* readily when necessary. *Unhealthy attitude systems* are *internally* full of *conflict* and do not accurately *correspond* to circumstances, leading to *experiences* of *frustration, failure*, and *alienation*. *Efforts* to cope with or *evade* these *feelings* tend to be both *self-perpetuating* and *self-defeating*, resulting in cumulative, *adaptational difficulties*.

Now let us look at the causation implied here. The goal of psychotherapy is to reduce distress (abstract) and improve functioning (which could be concrete potentially if we knew what it was). But to do this (here comes the start of a bigger story) we must change a person's *attitudes*, which we cannot observe and are hidden inside them. These attitudes *are affected by* (does this mean causation?) *emotional states* but which are also hidden and abstract. *Healthy attitudes* are *consistent* and *reflect reality* and these lead to a bunch of hidden and unobservable internals: "lead to *reliable, satisfactory* social interactions, accompanied by a *sense* of *competence, inner security*, and *well-being*". (This whole sentence is also probably a tautology except we cannot observe enough of the mentalistic components to decide.) Unhealthy attitudes lead to (cause?) a bunch of negative hidden and unobservable internals: "*experiences* of *frustration, failure*, and *alienation*".

Do you get the sense of word games taking place here? And this is an example from a good book! But remember what I wrote in Chapter 2. My approach to doing this based on my experience is the following:

- observe therapists and take what you see seriously
- listen to them talk *about what they actually do* and take this seriously, except when they use any abstract language
- *ignore how they explain what they do or why they do it*
- do not let the second two points put you off doing the first
- all 'therapies' have multiple component events occurring, any one of which could be what is causing the change, and not what the therapist is saying makes the change occur (Chapter 5)

The Frank paragraph above is a good example of this. There are some concrete foundations to what Frank is writing here, it is not gibberish, but everything is apparently caused within some hidden 'internal' world which is unobservable. The person's behaviour and their distress *are caused by these hidden attitudes not by the bad life situations they are trying to survive.* So, the bad life situations have been turned magically into *internal constructs* which we cannot see, and the job of psychotherapists becomes one of changing these hidden internal 'states', *rather than changing the bad life situations* (remember Figures 1.1, 1.2, and 1.3).

This chapter will have many more examples of similar explanations. The trick will be to see that these 'internal' states, experiences, attitudes, and consciousness are really about uses of *language*—how the person talks and thinks—and they are shaped by our external social world of conversation and discourses and can be observed, as it turns out. And what I hope to show is that when you remove all these fictitious stories, the multitude of therapies are really saying and doing the same things as each other! The differences are only in the words and stories they spin.

The plan for the next three chapters

I will cover several main points over the next three chapters. The rest of this chapter will continue to look in more detail at what therapists have *said* about what they do but treating this as discourse and not as a pure independent report of their observations. Chapter 4 will then look at the *methods of interventions* used by therapists, while Chapter 5 will look more loosely at *how therapists treat and interact with their recipients*; the more micro components of what they do, and how do they respond to the human being sitting in front of them.

For each of these chapters I will look at the question in several different ways, or from several different angles. The goal here is to explore what is going on in the therapy context, not just the background contexts we saw in Chapter 2 but more specifically.

Deconstructing 19 therapies to find the discursive goals of therapy and the material bases of change

Before commencing these micro-dissections of various aspects of therapy, I will describe one of the methods used, and then give some results spread over this chapter (talking about) and the next (doing). As a first attempt at looking more closely at the components of therapies, I studied 19 of the most common psychotherapies (Box 3.1; Guerin, 2017a). I reviewed the different forms of 19 psychological therapies and extracted what they each reported to be (1) *the discursive goals of the therapy* (this chapter), and (2) *the material activities carried out to achieve these goals* (the next chapter).

Box 3.1 The 19 psychotherapies reviewed plus others consulted

Psychoanalysis
Jungian Analysis
Adlerian Therapy
Existential Therapy
Person-Centered Therapy
Gestalt Therapy
Behaviour Therapy
Acceptance and Commitment Therapy
Dialectical Behaviour Therapy
Rational Emotive Behaviour Therapy
Beck Cognitive Therapy
Behavioural Activation Therapy
Mindfulness-Based Cognitive Therapy
Schema-Focused Therapy
Reality Therapy
Solution-Focused Therapy
Personal Construct Therapy
Narrative Therapy
Feminist Therapy
Tree hugging therapy (Chapter 5)
Star watching therapy (Chapter 5)

Other therapies consulted

Hypnosis
Pressure Method
Suggestion
Psychodrama (Role Reversal, Double Technique, Mirror Technique)
Art Therapy
Dance Movement Therapy
Drama Therapy
Music Therapy

To do this, I initially followed two standard textbooks, Sharf (2016) and Corsini and Wedding (2010). After this, dozens more psychotherapy textbooks were read but these proved to be mostly repetitions, and just a few extra new goals and therapeutic activities were included. To further explore the actual *activities* within the therapies, individual books, written by the therapists themselves where possible, were mined for descriptions and verbatim transcripts of actual therapies in practice (Chapter 4). Finally, many DVDs of the original therapists performing their therapies were watched for the techniques to be mentioned. In this way, the more concrete activities they actually used could be clarified.

Remember that these are what therapists report are their goals (this chapter) and what they report they do (Chapter 4). In Chapter 5, I will then look at other common components of what therapists do which were missed out in the *self-reported descriptions* of Chapters 3 and 4. That is, in Chapter 5 we will look at what might be happening in normal therapies that the therapist is not aware of, but which might better explain why they have some successes. I will include my own tree-hugging and star watching therapies in this.

As mentioned above, there was no illusion of being exhaustive for either the number of therapies or the goals and activities they use. Only the 19 main reported therapies were examined closely, and only the main reported goals and activities used for each of those therapies was noted. It should be clear, therefore, that this is not meant to be an exhaustive literature review but a springboard from which other therapies and techniques can be examined as well as missing components of the therapies (Chapter 5). Moreover, a point that will be noted below is that there was a lot of overlap in the activities found across the different therapies, even when therapies were trying to differentiate (or market) themselves as unique (in their talk), so being exhaustive would be fruitless. Also of note, the numerous forms of family therapy were left out since they required a more dedicated outline.

One big obstacle to this process was the language and jargon used by the different therapists, usually just repeated in the textbooks with some attempts at clarification (mainly by using more abstract words). It was at these points of abstract descriptions and jargon that specialist books and DVDs on the individual therapies were consulted. The techniques were then put into a more concrete form not reliant on any theoretical system. Basically, a description was attempted of those activities *which actually took place* in the therapeutic setting regardless of the language used by the authors to describe such events and their effects.

For the analyses presented here and in the next chapter, I grouped the *goals* and the *therapeutic activities* in various ways to show some patterns. These are certainly not meant as the only ways this can be done, and the full tables are provided so that readers can explore their own categorizations. The aim here was an attempt to explore mainly the convergences between stated goals and activities and, more particularly, the *functional* similarities.

Overall, it must again be repeated that doing this was not intended as some sort of 'proof' of what really takes place in therapy, nor an exhaustive catalogue of the verbal goals and techniques of therapy. There are too many gaps which preclude this, and I have just listed many of these gaps above. In fact, such a purpose would be futile in any case because therapies constantly change and adapt, and they borrow from each other. There are also many nuances that cannot be captured in the process carried out here, since they cannot be easily 'described' in words, especially when I was comparing what was theorized to what was seen in the DVDs. I was keenly aware that the therapies were all much more similar in the DVDs than in any of the discourses surrounding what is done and with what verbalized goals. It is when you watch the therapies in action that you can see how similar they really are.

The aim, then, of this methodology was to find a way to describe therapies as concrete activities which take place within limited social contexts (Chapter 2)—stripped of all the words, marketing, and theories spun around them. It was hoped that the ideas stemming from this, while not in any way proof of another better system of therapy, would be useful. In the terms used by many of these same therapies, the purpose was to find a concrete process to 'reframe', 'socially reconstruct' or 're-story' the way therapies are thought about, studied, and practised. The aim was certainly not to find the ultimate therapy by combining all these!

A first approach to 'What therapists say': the discourses spun around the 19 psychotherapies

Deciphering the stated 'goals'

Table 3.1 shows the main goals as expressed by each of the 19 therapies. As can be seen, these are replete with jargon, metaphors and storied foundations. I will help decipher these shortly since having jargon does not mean that they are fictitious. We just need to contextualize the jargon.

So, the first step to deconstructing the therapies is to look at these verbal goals as expressed and then read up on them and get an understanding of what these varied and often colourful words and stories really mean in concrete terms. The next step was to look for the common ideas, discourses or ways of talking across all the therapies (Chapter 1). While not using the exact same words in their writings, *most of the reported goals are really saying the same thing in different words*. Table 3.2 presents one attempt to group these. I have listed the common phrases used to state and justify the goals of therapy and put them into 11 categories (my headings) plus some uncategorized.

As an example, 'reality' is used in the discourses of several therapies usually to describe a common idea that 'people have different versions of reality' which needs to be taken into account when solving social disputes and 'misperceptions'. Others use the same word 'reality' to say that what is important is how people 'perceive' their own reality (which no one else can know, they claim),

Table 3.1 The reported goals of therapy as reported for 19 types of therapy. Therapies later in this list often include goals mentioned earlier but these are not repeated. For example, Jungian analysis includes many of the same goals as psychoanalysis. This highlights the similarities between all these therapies.

Type of therapy	Goals
Psychoanalysis	Changes in personality and character structure Understanding unconscious material (especially sexual and aggressive drives, ego defence, relationships with self and other especially separation issues) Resolve unconscious conflicts Self-understanding of childhood experiences Feel more authentic or real
Jungian Analysis	Individuation Integrate conscious and unconscious parts of self
Adlerian Therapy	Change self-defeating behaviours and improve problem-solving Increase social interest and sense of belonging Primarily motived by social relations not sexual urges Finding mistaken goals and faulty assumptions
Existential Therapy	Authenticity Develop purpose Recognize self-deception Experience existence as real Face anxieties and fears
Person-Centered Therapy	Move away from phoniness and superficiality Openness to experience Trusting of self (be 'true' self) More self-directed Not solve problems but foster independence and integration
Gestalt Therapy	Mature and grow, foster growth Take self-responsibly Can do more than they think they can Self-awareness Self-actualization Be here-and-now Integrate feelings, perceptions, thoughts, and body processes Resolve unfinished business
Behaviour Therapy	Specific goals, target behaviours Functional analysis Change behaviours Insight not needed New goals
Acceptance and Commitment Therapy	Using language to alleviate distress Reduce avoidance of feelings and thoughts Treat thoughts as words and not own them Creative hopelessness, to be open to suggestions Cognitive diffusion

Type of therapy	Goals
Dialectical Behaviour Therapy	Balance acceptance and change Persuade to try new change methods (dialectic) Accept emotions and experiences and change
Rational Emotive Behaviour Therapy	Minimize emotional disturbances Decrease self-defeating self-behaviours More self-actualized Think more rationally Feel more appropriately Act more efficiently and effectively
Behavioural Activation Therapy	Develop routines and activities Modify environments rather than thinking Deal with avoidance activities
Beck Cognitive Therapy	Remove biases and distortions from their thinking Challenge the thinking Short term specific goals
Mindfulness-Based Cognitive Therapy	Separating thoughts from reality Change way of attending to negative thoughts Change attention for other parts of life
Schema-Focused Therapy	Identify and change distorted thinking schema Attend to childhood for schema origins
Reality Therapy	Help people meet psychological needs for survival, belonging, power, freedom, and fun Get realistic goals Educate about how to achieve
Solution-Focused Therapy	Find how the person views their problems Focus on solution instead of reasons or origin Small changes Have clear goals
Personal Construct Therapy	Focus on stories about problems Change or modify the stories Analyze like a drama, novel or play
Narrative Therapy	Attend to stories Re-author the stories Make problem a character Write solutions into stories Make stories positive
Feminist Therapy	Changing the life, not adjusting Improving the client's nurturance and self-esteem Changing society also, committing to social change Empowerment Diversity Body image Balance instrumental and relationship goals Cultural analysis Gender analysis

Table 3.2 My categorization of some terms used by therapists to describe their goals of therapy. The labels are mine, but the words are those used by therapists to state their goals.

Categories	Therapists' goals
Reality	Reality not observable
	Thinking is not reality
	Everyone's reality is different
	Everything social constructed
	Cannot know reality
	We all use different constructs to view the world
	Realities are socially constructed
	We live our lives with stories
	Perceptions of reality important for understanding people
	Subjective reality
	Subjectivity
	Perceived meaning
Logic/rational/dialectic/ persuasion	Logic and dialectic
	Existence opposite to rationality
	Irrationality
	Functional and non-functional
Consciousness/subjectivity	Consciousness
	Perception
	Internal dialogue
Unconscious	Unconscious
	Unconscious = external context, the social relationship context of language
	Unconscious motivations
	Collective unconscious
	Archetypes
	Dreams
Mind/mental/internalizing	Mind
	Mental
	Internalizing
Self/authenticity	Self-actualization
	Authenticity
	Genuineness
	Self/ego/identity
	Being-in-the-world
Self-control	Self-efficacy
	Self-control
	Self-instruction
Cognitive processes/defence mechanisms	Defence mechanisms
	Cognitive defusion
	Cognitive distortions
	Automatic thoughts
	Core beliefs
	Schema
	Projection
	Resistance
	Repression
	Unfinished business

Categories	Therapists' goals
Resources	Needs
	Motivations
	Repressed instincts
	Reinforcements
	Punishments
Social relationships	Transference
	Attachment
	Empathy
	Unconditional positive regard
Thinking and doing	Being-oneself (language) and Being-there which is direct (doing)
	Congruent
	Externalizing
	Mindfulness
Other	Personality
	Performative
	Choice
	Acceptance
	Shaping
	Behavioural activation
	Guided imagery
	Modelling
	Emotions

as opposed to some 'objective reality'. Still others use it to argue that we can all have differing conceptions of 'reality' and that is okay; you are okay if your version of events differs from someone else's (presumably so long as it does not involve murder or mayhem!). These are all used to explain or justify the therapies in question.

As can be seen in Table 3.2, there are several key terms used to describe the goals of therapy but notice how abstract and ambiguous these terms are. Hardly a solid foundation to a 'science'. My next aim is not to discredit these, but to show how we can get a more concrete list which includes the external observable contexts for these and stops them being just vague, abstract and ambiguous words spun into theoretical and marketable stories. To do this we need to continue what was briefly begun at the end of Chapter 1 and will be continued in Chapters 6 and 7. To make a more concrete sense of these highly abstract words which are only pretending to explain anything as they are currently found.

Translating the jargon into contextual terms

For this discussion I will try to present a social contextual or behavioural analysis version, even though each point will not get full agreement from all readers (Chapters 6 and 7; Guerin, 2016). As mentioned, readers are welcome to find other ways to make these terms more concrete and then to try other analyses. Any method of putting what is said to go on in therapy into context and into more concrete terms beyond jargon will be useful. These can be added to the ones at the end of Chapter 1.

Reality: In contextual terms, when these reported goals are put into more observable forms, they appear to mean that the person's *words* are not matching what is happening with their contingent relations (social and non-social), so the goal of therapy is to match their verbal behaviour more closely with what is shaping them in their world, or to try talking about their world in new ways. As these goals are stated, this could mean trying to prevent verbal constructions of their world, shaping new ways to talk about their world, or giving them skills to gauge their verbal constructions.

Logic/rational/dialectic/persuasion: These goals seem to be giving the client (persuading or forcing them really) new ways to talk and act, which are apparently more functional in terms of everyday life, or more logical or rational (which is really only useful to persuade other people in their lives).

Consciousness/subjectivity: These goals aim to have clients be able to verbalize about their language use or their behaviour. Assisting them to become more conscious probably comes close to some forms of mindfulness training, meaning that they are able to verbalize or experience more of what is being done or said and the consequences of these actions or words.

Unconscious: Making the person's unconscious thoughts or wishes conscious is a goal in many therapies. In more concrete terms, this usually refers to learning how to name or to talk about those external life contingences shaping their behaviour which the person could not previously name or is 'unaware'. Different therapies are referring to local social relationships shaping the person's behaviour (which they are not conscious of, meaning they cannot talk about it), and also the societal forces shaping a person's behaviour (such as patriarchy in feminist therapies; and others hidden in the jargon, Guerin, 2019).

Mind/mental/internalizing: Many of the therapy goals refer to changing or influencing mental or mind contents which are said to be internal to the person (Chapter 1). A contextual description would be that these refer to external shapers which are difficult to observe or notice (Chapter 6), and in particular they are likely to be social or discursive contexts. Suggestions have been made elsewhere for how to translate many of the specific cognitive or mental descriptions into descriptions based on observable discourse analysis or behaviour analysis (Guerin, 2016, 2017b, 2020b).

Self/authenticity: The goal of building a strong sense of self or authenticity usually refers to socially shaping *stories* which a person can maintain about themselves in their real social communities, and which are hopefully beneficial to them. To become *authentic* might also sometimes refer to aligning what a person says about themselves and what they do, in a similar way to the 'reality' goals given above. The reader can hopefully see how even the disparate-looking existential and narrative therapies converge when framed in this way.

Self-control: This group of reported goals probably concerns aligning what is said and what is done in a way to increase the following of 'self-statements'. In a contextual analysis, the 'self' statements are shaped by external audiences, so in concrete terms the therapist probably shapes the client to both say new things about themselves and what they will do, and also to follow those statement descriptions (which will still need audience control, but the therapist is assumed to be a strong audience). In terms of later tables, these might be specific, local changes or else broader life changes and values.

Cognitive processes/defence mechanisms: These are goals to do with shaping all the language behaviours, primarily those done by the therapist as the audience. Some are about stopping language behaviours (changing cognitive distortions or dysfunctional cognitions; cognitive defusion), and some about changing common language behaviours which are used by clients to shape their own audiences (defence mechanisms, resistance, and core beliefs converge here). Both the 'cognition' and the 'unconscious defence mechanisms' are, in more observable terms, language behaviours shaped by the clients' external and concrete interactions with audiences.

Resources: These are the things or events in life by which the external environment has shaped behaviour, and for therapy, these involve the normal audiences of the client and their roles in the client's life. Some are probably more about the verbal descriptions of possible resources than about actually engaging with those resources.

Social relationships: These goal areas are about shaping social relationships in all their complexity, either with the therapist for therapeutic outcomes (transference, unconditional positive regard) or with other people in the client's life.

Thinking and doing: Like authenticity as a goal, these are goals to (re)shape the person's language behaviour with respect to their other actions.

Meaning: The term 'meaning' was not directly used in Table 3.2 but is a commonly used term and, once again, is very abstract and metaphorical. Titchener put it well: "meaning, psychologically, is always context" (1921, p. 367). But this still does not tell us what parts of a person's 'contexts' is their 'meaning', and further exploration with the person is always needed *to translate meaning into something more concrete in their life*. What someone calls 'meaning' could be their long-term life plans and dreams (discourses); it could be the hidden conflicts and social relationship disputes behind some event or action they have done; or in terms of 'I want to do something meaningful' it could be finding new discourses of a way forward or a path involving other people in new resources and new friendships or admiration. This can also be reflected in comments about people 'searching for meaning'. So, once again, the idea is not to dismiss the use of the words as empty, but to explore further with the person the more concrete substance of the term.

Commonalities of the discursive goals of therapy

From the analysis so far, we can see that the talking about therapy is very abstract and ambiguous. When we try and put the talking into more concrete contexts, it turns out that most of what is said is about ways to change what a person is saying—changing their discursive contexts in some ways. This is the major stated goal of therapy when the abstractions are 'translated' into concrete contexts, along with fixing problems for the person.

The next step after contextualizing all the main concepts given in Table 3.2 (above) for the goals of therapy, was to gather together all the now contextualized goals which were basically the same but had used different jargon. Box 3.2 shows the main headings once all the many goals are together.

Box 3.2 Functional or contextualized groups of contextualized therapy goals

Practical/ Problem solving/ Specific behaviours

Resources
Social relationships

Practical life issues/ General behaviour patterns

Resources
Social relationships

Changing talking and thinking

About self
About social relationships
Changing the talk itself

So, the main divisions of therapeutic goals are between (1) dealing with specific or local problems in the person's life, (2) more general of life problems in the person's life, and (3) attempting to change the way the person talks and thinks. When we get to the next chapter, we will see that these actually mirror what therapists do in therapy, once those therapeutic goals are put into concrete terms. Most are based on methods using talk and changing discourses (with the therapist acting as a new discursive community).

Table 3.3 shows the full detail of this grouping of the basic goals of the 19 therapies.

In contextualizing these, it must be remembered that resources and social relationships will always be entwined (Guerin, 2020a), and that 'talking and thinking about self' is really also about social relationships (Guerin, 2020c). To contextualize further, the 'general life problems' will usually refer to those situations shaped not by single other people, but by societal or group shaping.

We can now begin to get an idea of what the 19 therapies *say* they are trying to achieve. Some focus more in individual and local problems for the client (e.g., solution-based), others on broader problems (e.g., dialectical behaviour therapy), and some on how people are talking and thinking about their lives and societal shaping out of their control (e.g., existential therapy). And despite

Table 3.3 One way of reframing the reported goals of therapies in Table 3.1 into three functional groups

1. Practical/ Problem solving/ Dealing with specific behaviours

Resources

Change self-defeating behaviours and improve problem-solving
Can do more than they think they can
Specific goals, target behaviours
Functional analysis
Change behaviours
Act more efficiently and effectively
Short term specific goals
Help people meet psychological needs for survival, belonging, power, freedom, and fun
Educate about how to achieve
Find how the person views their problems
Focus on solution instead of reasons or origin
Small changes
Set goals
Meet individual and family needs
Concrete goals

Relationships

Increase social interest and sense of belonging
Deal with avoidance activities
Reduce family stress and conflict
Listen to family dynamics
Family choosing goals to reduce anxiety

2. Practical life issues/ Dealing with general behaviour patterns

Resources

Changes in personality and character structure
Understanding unconscious material (especially sexual and aggressive drives, ego defense, relationships with self and other especially separation issues)
Resolve unconscious conflicts
Finding mistaken goals and faulty assumptions
Openness to experience
Mature and grow, foster growth
Integrate feelings, perceptions, thoughts, and body processes
Balance acceptance and change
Develop routines and activities
Modify environments rather than thinking
Changing the life, not adjusting
Changing society also, committing to social change
Empowerment

Relationships

Primarily motived by social relations not sexual urges
Not solve problems but foster independence and integration
Balance instrumental and relationship goals
Cultural analysis
Gender analysis

3. Changing talking and thinking

About self

Self-understanding of childhood experiences
Feel more authentic or real
Integrate conscious and unconscious parts of self
Develop purpose
Recognize self-deception
Face anxieties and fears
Trusting of self (be 'true' self)
Take self-responsibly
Self-awareness
New goals
Decrease self-defeating self-behaviours
Attend to childhood for schema origins
Get realistic goals
Have clear goals
Improving the client's nurturance and self-esteem
Body image
Authenticity
More self-directed
Self-actualization
More self-actualized

About relationships

Move away from phoniness and superficiality
Resolve unfinished business
Accept emotions and experiences and change
Minimize emotional disturbances
Feel more appropriately

Changing the talk itself

Individuation
Experience existence as real
Be here-and-now
Using language to alleviate distress
Reduce avoidance of feelings and thoughts
Treat thoughts as words and not own them
Creative hopelessness, to be open to suggestions
Cognitive defusion
Persuade to try new change methods (dialectic)
Think more rationally
Remove biases and distortions from their thinking
Challenge the thinking
Separating thoughts from reality
Change way of attending to negative thoughts
Change attention for other parts of life
Identify and change distorted thinking schema
Focus on stories about problems
Change or modify the stories
Analyse like a drama, novel or play
Attend to stories
Re-author the stories
Make problem a character
Write solutions into stories
Make stories positive

the plethora of different-looking words, there are similar goals across all 19, once you contextualize the words they are using to describe what they are trying to achieve, and realize that *most therapies are trying to change recipients' discourses by using discourses*. And most of the therapies are really using different jargons and stories to account for the same three main goals of therapy.

A second approach to 'What therapists say': the DSM, formulations, and contextual analyses

Another way to glimpse how therapists talk about therapy is to look at how they talk and write about 'cases'. How do they summarize the outcomes of therapy? There are many forms of this, but they can give us some clues about the differences between therapies, other than the theoretical reports of therapists about what they do, seen in the tables above.

'Case notes'

The obvious source on how therapists talk about therapy would come from the 'case notes' made by psychiatrists, psychologists, and other therapists during and after sessions of therapy. Unfortunately, these are normally considered confidential; even, in the case of much psychiatry, confidential from the client themselves.

A few examples are known through some clients who have managed to gain access in different ways. A person I know had been asking their psychiatrist not to be given certain psychiatric drugs based on their previous experiences. They happened later to see the notes made by the psychiatrist that day, and it had 'oppositional' written on it. In some parts of the world, privacy laws should make such notes available to recipients of therapy at least, but the power differentials and discursive dominance of the therapist (Chapter 2) usually means that recipients do not even try.

DSM

Much of the talking about therapy disappeared when the DSM was introduced (1952; APA, 2013). This categorization system focused therapy very narrowly on reaching a diagnosis in a vast and changing category system, and this DSM-talk is generally a large part of conversations about clients now. I have been present in many such conversations and they are focused almost exclusively on *getting to a diagnosis* – since the medical model is that once you get the right diagnosis you will have the appropriate treatment. As we saw in Chapter 1, this is fiction in the 'mental health' arena.

A major problem is that once a diagnosis is reached, however tentatively, further contextual information is generally not sought, and discussion usually stops. So, the DSM labels have come to act as a sort of shorthand way of talking about a person and their life history. They are now the standard way of talking about and making inferences about clients, therapy goals, and any issues arising.

Biology and zoology do a similar thing to the medical model, but when you have identified the genus and species of an animal you are observing, you can indeed know a lot about the science of this animal's life, physiology and even ecology (Guerin, 2017b). Given this, the DSM would not be so bad except that the 'science' is missing, and the category system is based on judgements of a team of psychiatrists using their personal 'knowledge' and experience (Bentall, 2006; Caplan, 1995; Davies, 2014; Guerin, 2020b; Johnstone, 2014; Johnstone & Boyle, 2018; Kinderman, 2019; Watson, 2019). They even *voted* for the placements of categories amongst their group, given there was no science behind it. So, learning a person's diagnosis does not help either to understand what the person is going through, nor is it a guide to what specific treatments are linked to diagnoses, again unlike general medicine.

The DSM is hopefully on its way out, and criticism has been mounting over the last decade (Adame, 2014; Blackburn, 2021; Moncrieff, 2010). The main argument in defence currently seems to be, "Well, what are you going to do instead? There are no alternatives". Luckily, there *are* alternatives, and many therapy clinics are now operating successfully without any diagnosis using the DSM (Guerin, 2020b; Johnstone & Boyle, 2018). Unfortunately, government systems are wedded to the DSM because it assists in the neoliberal processing of 'cases'. (Even zoology has alternatives to the Linnaeus system of animal categories, such as cladistics.)

> ... it does mean that it is no longer scientifically, professionally or ethically justifiable to insist on psychiatric diagnosis as *the only way of describing* people's distress. If the authors of the diagnostic manuals are admitting that the diagnoses are not supported by evidence and that the process of developing them is 'not scientific', *then no one should be forced to accept them.*
>
> (Johnstone, 2014, p. 17. First italics mine.)

So, the DSM has been a strong inhibitor of how therapists and others talk about people in distress, and has narrowed all our discourses. Part of this book's aims is to broaden the discourses around people in distress and find new ways to talk, other than the throttling effects of the DSM, about understanding people in distress.

Traditional formulations in psychology and psychiatry

Another form of therapists' writings and discourses about therapy and recipients is 'formulations'. These are often compiled from case notes but form a summary of the 'case' and ways forward (Johnstone & Dallos, 2014). There are many different types of formulations and, of more importance here, many different ways of writing them and involving the clients (or not). Some very traditional examples are given in Sperry (1992), and Slysz and Soroko (2021) give some examples of constructing case conceptualizations. Johnstone and Dallos (2014) is the best source.

The problem with formulations traditionally is that they have incorporated the therapist's theories or world views *into the formulation itself.* They can emphasize the biological, the psychoanalytic, the behavioural, the biopsychosocial viewpoints, or even cultural elements (La Roche & Bloom, 2018), although most formulations are now principally discussions of how DSM categories apply to the person. But this means that the recommended way forward (usually a form of treatment) is dependent upon the practitioner's stance on things (Joseph, 2021). This shows in the different versions: psychiatric, psychological, cognitive-behaviour therapy (Persons, 2008), and even for children (La Roche & Bloom, 2018).

So, the main criticisms have been about incorporating theoretical notions (including a heavy dose of DSM) into formulations but then acting as if they were independent, 'objective', 'scientific', etc. (Joseph, 2021) when they are not. Dembo and Hanfmann (1935) provide some early research as witnesses to when some 'clients' admitted to an asylum first read the 'superintendent's letter' which was the early equivalent of a formulation, constructed unilaterally by the admitting psychiatrist after a very short interview. Most clients were very upset and normally left alone to read it. Many of their subsequent 'pathological' behaviours were actually due to reading the contents of this letter.

Newer approaches to 'formulations'

There have been recent attempts not only to change the DSM (preferably remove its use altogether and just look at behaviours) but also to use new forms of formulations (Ball & Ritchie, 2021; Boyle & Johnstone, 2020; Johnstone, 2018; Johnstone & Dallos, 2014; La Roche & Bloom, 2018; Randall, Johnson & Johnstone, 2020). The new forms are trying these new features:

- having the 'client' participate in formulating and writing the formulation
- making it more like a life narrative than a 'factual' account
- constantly revising the formulation, with the client participating, rather than producing one 'definitive' account
- having the client write their own 'self-formulation'
- sharing the editing and writing of the person's 'construct'
- adding more effects of society such as economic disadvantage, culture, and patriarchy (Power Threat Meaning Framework)

So basically, formulations are including a lot more details of the person's history and life, and removing the categorical summations, as well as involving the persons themselves in all this reporting.

Social Contextual Analyses

For many years, most of my research has been exploring with people the many contexts that shape what they do, that have shaped their lives, and trying to describe these. This is heavily based on the contextual approaches in social anthropology research, sociology, sociolinguistics, and discourse analysis. More recently this has included people who have at some time received DSM labels as 'explanations' for what they do. In this research we explore all the social relationships, cultural, economic, patriarchal, historical, and other contexts that have shaped their current behaviours, and the Resource-Social Relationship pathways they are on (Guerin, 2016b, 2020b).

A side-effect of doing this is that many of the people in these research projects have later remarked that they have learned so much about themselves which was unknown to them, as one might expect. But more than this, despite doing such exploration as research and therefore without any thought of this changing the person or being a form of therapy, many people report that it had helped them in a more therapeutic way and led them to make some changes in their life and social relationships.

This prompted three thoughts for me:

- that just exploring what has been, and is, controlling and shaping your behaviours (and life) can help people with their life 'problems' and issues as well
- that this is part of the power of *good* formulations when they are done collaboratively, and they cover a large numbers of life contexts (Boyle & Johnstone, 2020)
- maybe this is also partly what a lot of therapies probably do, sometimes inadvertently when getting the person to 'explore their feelings' and do other language responses within all the different variants of therapy

This reminded me, curiously, of people I have known who really study Karl Marx properly and say that it has helped them understand their own life, since they began to see how societal contexts (mainly economic ones) have shaped their lives and the people before them. And this also appears 'therapeutic' to many of them. It also appears in a report on how war veterans *doing activism work* began to learn about the bigger picture and how they had been shaped (Schrader, 2019) and how this affected them. Feminist therapy also reports a similar idea, urging women in therapy to become engaged in women's rights and activism, and begin to see how the forces that have shaped their lives are not their own fault but are ingrained in societal patriarchies. And importantly, feminist therapists report that even though the women cannot then smash the patriarchy, *just learning and exploring these contexts in terms of their own lives* is already therapeutic for them.

> I worked with a young woman from Guatemala over twenty years ago who struggled with suicide and substance abuse. She had been told she would be in psychotherapy for the rest of her life given the extent of the political violence she had suffered. She thought I was a pretty good therapist. Eventually, this young survivor grew frustrated with other professional helpers and foster parents telling her she should stay alone, study,

and journal. She resisted this professional advice and participated in the Theatre of the Oppressed with fifty other refugee youths, some of them children and grandchildren of the disappeared, who create political theatre together in Spanish. I asked a question from Australian narrative therapist Michael White; 'You've said our sessions are pretty good. How many sessions do you think one political activity was worth?' She reflected a bit and said tentatively, 'Probably over a hundred.' I hold this humbling teaching close: a spirited activist event can be worth a hundred therapy sessions.

(Reynolds, 2016, p. 183)

This also links to accounts of people themselves in therapy beginning their own contextual analysis of their life either through bibliotherapy routes or because once having accepted that some change is needed, they begin to think and remember more honestly (accurately). This is echoed in the following:

I had many patients write a letter to me, explain that they want help … and not mail it … they went through that formal conscious process of asking for help and then their unconscious would answer them. So when I am just a memory, you will write to me and your unconscious can answer your letter.

Milton H. Erickson (1974)

The point of this is that, as will be mentioned again in Chapter 5, just recognizing that they require help is often by itself enough to begin this exploration, regardless of whether therapy actually then occurs. People can explore their own external contextual worlds (a.k.a. the 'unconscious') and do the changes by themselves.

The upshot of these examples is that having people explore their own life contexts, and what local and societal forces have shaped them into the position they are now in, seems by itself to be 'therapeutic'; whether this happens as part of a formal therapy or not. *The DSM constricts exploration of a person's life world*, whereas newer forms of formulation, constructs, and social contextual analyses begin to show people what has shaped their world and behaviour, and how they might go about trying to change this. Purely referring to the problems as 'in your head' goes around and around in storied circles and puts the blame on them, though there is no reduction of suffering. This seems to be especially important when the contexts shaping the behaviours are difficult to observe: discourses shaped by societal discursive communities; societal forces such as arise from the consequences of economic, patriarchal, and colonizing forces; and social relationship power imbalances (Guerin, 2020a; Johnstone & Boyle, 2018).

References

Adame, A. L. (2014). "There needs to be a place in society for madness": The Psychiatric Survivor Movement and new directions in mental health care. *Journal of Humanistic Psychology*, 54, 456–475.

American Psychiatric Association (2013). *The diagnostic and statistical manual of mental disorders* (5th Ed.). Washington: APA.

Ball, M. & Ritchie, R. (2021). *Suicide narratives: Healing through knowing*. www.humaneclinic.com.au/suicide-narratives?fbclid=IwAR0wLVo402gTWDZW1LHoNAU6uPe2ogsQB4MQNM8SfYrLiUy-P2xkBv3XByw.

Bentall, R. P. (2006). Madness explained: Why we must reject the Kraepelinian paradigm and replace it with a 'complaint-orientated' approach to understanding mental illness. *Medical Hypotheses*, 66, 220–233.

Blackburn, P. (2021). *The ERNI Declaration: Making sense of distress without 'disease'*. Sourced: www.madinamerica.com/2021/05/erni-declaration/?fbclid=IwAR1IXgFno8ufUy8KPvzWikK7hO9gMlN8p3fv0gPpDA5VdZdH3TrOVyNOESw.

Boyle, M. & Johnstone, L. (2020). *A straight talking introduction to the Power Meaning Threat Framework: An alternative to psychiatric diagnosis*. Monmouth: PCCS Books.

Caplan, P. J. (1995). *They say you're crazy: How the world's most powerful psychiatrists decide who's normal*. NY: Life Long.

Corsini, R. J., & Wedding, D. (2010). *Current psychotherapies* (9th Ed). NY: Brooks/Cole.

Davies, J. (2014). *Cracked: Why psychiatry is doing more harm than good*. London: Icon Books.

Dembo, T., & Hanfmann, E. (1935). The patient's psychological situation upon admission to a mental hospital. *American Journal of Psychology*, 47, 381–408.

Erickson, M. H. (1974). *Quoted in Principles and core competencies of Ericksonian therapy*, 2019 edition.

Frank, J. D. (1975). *Persuasion and healing: A comparative study of psychotherapy*. NY: Schocken Books.

Guerin, B. (2016a). *How to rethink psychology: New metaphors for understanding people and their behavior*. London: Routledge.

Guerin, B. (2016b). *How to rethink human behavior: A practical guide to social contextual analysis*. London: Routledge.

Guerin, B. (2017a). Deconstructing psychological therapies as activities in context: What are the goals and what do therapists actually do? *Revista Perspectivas em Análise do Comportamento*, 8, 97–119.

Guerin, B. (2017b). *How to rethink mental illness: The human contexts behind the labels*. London: Routledge.

Guerin, B. (2019). What do therapists and clients talk about when they cannot explain behaviours? How Carl Jung avoided analysing a client's environments by inventing theories. *Revista Perspectivas em Anályse Comportamento*, 10, 76–97.

Guerin, B. (2020a). *Turning psychology into social contextual analysis*. London: Routledge.

Guerin, B. (2020b). *Turning mental health into social action*. London: Routledge.

Guerin, B. (2020c). *Turning psychology into a social science*. London: Routledge.

Johnstone, L. (2014). *A straight talking introduction to psychiatric diagnosis*. London: PCCS Books.

Johnstone, L. (2018). Psychological formulation as an alternative to psychiatric diagnosis. *Journal of Humanist Psychology*, 58, 30–46.

Johnstone, L., Boyle, M., Cromby, J., Dillon, J., Harper, D., Kinderman, P., … Read, J. (2018). *The Power Threat Meaning Framework: Towards the identification of patterns in emotional distress, unusual experiences and troubled or troubling behaviour, as an alternative to functional psychiatric diagnosis*. Leicester: British Psychological Society.

Johnstone, L., & Dallos, R. (Eds.). (2014). *Formulation in psychology and psychotherapy*. London: Routledge.

Joseph, S. (2021). Psychological formulation, a critical viewpoint: Illness ideology in disguise. *Journal of Humanist Psychology*, 60, 1–11.

Kinderman, P. (2019). *A manifesto for mental health: Why we need a revolution in mental health care*. London: Palgrave Macmillan.

La Roche, M. J., & Bloom, J. B. (2018). Examining the effectiveness of the Cultural Formulation Interview with young children: A clinical illustration. *Transcultural Psychiatry*, 45, 1–16.

Moncrieff, J. (2010). Psychiatric diagnosis as a political device. *Social Theory & Health*, 8, 370–382.

Persons, J. B. (2008). *The case formulation approach to cognitive-behavior therapy*. NY: Guildford Press.

Randall, J., Johnson, E. & Johnstone, L. (2020). Self-formulation: Making sense of your own experiences. In J. Randall (Ed.), *Surviving clinical psychology: Navigating personal, professional and political selves on the journey to qualification* (pp. 142–164). London: Routledge.

Reynolds, V. (2016). Hate kills. In J. White, I. Marsh, M. J. Kral, & J. Morris (Eds.), *Critical suicidology: Transforming suicide research and prevention for the 21st century* (pp. 169–187). Toronto: University of British Columbia Press.

Schrader, B. (2019). The affect of veteran activism. *Critical Military Studies*, 5, 63–77.

Sharf, R. S. (2016). *Theories of psychotherapy and counseling: Concepts and cases* (6th Ed.). Boston, MA: Cengage Learning.

Slysz, A., & Soroko, E. (2021). How do psychotherapists develop a case conceptualisation? Thematic analysis of conceptual maps. *Journal of Contemporary Psychotherapy*, 51, 87–96.

Sperry, L. (1992). Demystifying the psychiatric case formulation. *Jefferson Journal of Psychiatry*, 10, 12–19.

Titchener, E. B. (1921). *A text-book of psychology*. NY: Macmillan.

Watson, J. (2019). *Drop the disorder: Challenging the culture of psychiatric diagnosis*. London: PCCS Books.

4   What do therapists do, in general?

'Applying treatments' as a misleading metaphor

In this chapter I will dissect how some of the therapy approaches talk about dealing with people in 'mental health' distress. This will not have all the answers, primarily because contextual approaches assume that most of the bad life situations, and the behaviours which get shaped, are very idiosyncratic and not to be easily categorized or 'cured with a magic one-size-fits-all bullet'. That way of thinking needs to stop, such as when therapists claim to have a model that works for most people. This is not to say that they are *not* helpful sometimes, just that we do not need all the jargon and marketing wrapped around what does and does not work, to inflate these therapy approaches.

In the next chapter I will break some of the current 'treatments' into even more fine-grained components. The main point of doing this across both chapters is to show that *all therapies and methods of healing have very many components*, and no single mixture is going to work all the time, so all the theories and marketing are misplaced or misleading. Nor is it the case that all those therapies that work 'sometimes' must be sharing a single common 'magic bullet', since we saw in Chapter 2 that there are so many differential contexts which mould the very therapies themselves—it is not all about what the 'client' does. Those trying to help need to be sensitized so they can begin to observe all these components in action, and *be better attuned to what is going on for the person in front of them*, with all the surrounding contexts (Chapter 7). And trying to relate this to a category system of the 'usual' components of 'evidence-based' therapies is wasting time (since testing the 'evidence' requires specific restrictions on contextual features, which will not necessarily apply in the real world).

So, my whole aim here is to break up the standard chatter that (1) a person has problems, and (2) the source of the problems is inside the person, (3) so they come to see the therapist in an office, who (4) uses their skills to do some techniques with (or worse 'on') the person, which then (5) changes 'the person' or their behaviour and (6) helps them out. We need to break out of this mould, and I will come back to alternatives in the final chapters of this book.

In the previous chapter I looked at the stated goals of 19 of the major psychotherapies and below we will examine the reported *major activities* of these same 19 psychotherapies. What was most important was to strip away the jargon and talk used by the therapy itself, and instead look at the behaviours

DOI: 10.4324/9781003300571-5

carried out, the contexts in which they were carried out, and the outcomes. A second way of reimagining therapy and 'healing' is to look more at what is going on in the context of the client's life (Chapters 8 and 9). This requires new approaches in practice, however.

What we can glean from older therapies?

As a great start, I will briefly outline Pierre Janet's 1919 compendium of all the methods of 'healing' (Janet, 1925/1919; Janet, 1924). Like my approach, Janet also ignored most of the jargon and theories used by the therapists themselves and brought into focus (1) what was being done, (2) in what contexts, and (3) with what effects. For example, "Although, theoretically considered, Mrs. Eddy's doctrines may seem to be nothing more than those of a trite and very illogical idealism, the practical results of Christian Science are unrivalled, and give the philosophy the stamp of organizability." (Janet, 1925/1919, Vol. 1, p. 80). We might make the same comments on many current therapies (and I will in Chapter 10).

Janet also gives many examples for each method with reasonable descriptions of some of the context. What is most remarkable for this book is that most of the methods and techniques used in the 19 psychotherapies listed earlier, appear with different words in Janet's book from 1919. The same 'techniques', but talked about in different words.

Box 4.1 Gives Janet's main headings of therapies and healing with a brief indication of what was being done.

The main categories of therapy listed in Janet (1925/1919; 1924) with a brief description

Part 1. Search for mental and moral action

1. Miraculous healings

Janet looks here at religious miracles, magical miracles, and animal magnetism. He provides examples and then warns sceptics (in a similar way to Chapters 3 and 5) not to confuse the talking about miracles with what actually occurs, which sometimes seems to be an immediate change in behaviour. He concludes that better observations and more of the context is needed to say why some miracle cures seem to occur and exactly under what conditions, rather than believe the discourses that practitioners give or disbelieve without closer observations of the concrete events.

2. Philosophical methods of treatment

Janet outlines some rational, philosophical, and quasi-spiritual treatments where a philosophical (that is, discursive) change for the person seems to produce change. He goes through the Christian Science movement or church of Mary Baker Eddy, which produced healing through scriptures of behaviours we would now call 'mental health' as well as other types. The outline can also be compared to much older forms of philosophy in Greek and Roman times, but which were non-spiritual (e. g., Addiss, 2008; Fairbank, 1957; Hadot, 1995).

3. Medical moralization

Janet outlines Paul Dubois' methods of medical moralization (circa 1900). These basically were a philosophical way of persuading clients out of their symptoms (again, discursive changes). Dubois used a little hypnotism, but also suggestion and authority to persuade. Similar methods by Strümpell, Oppenheim, Jolly, Forel, and many more are also included. Janet's summary pretty much outlines modern cognitive approaches and its talk of 'faulty cognitive processing': "We shall understand our patients better when we realize that under the influence of erroneous ideas they have adopted a number of bad mental habits." (p. 105). And later, comparing the religious to non-religious versions, "The idea of 'error' is a vaguer one than that of 'sin'" (p. 128).

Part 2. Utilization of the patient's automatism

4. History of suggestion and hypnosis

5. Definition of suggestion

6. Conditions under which suggestion occurs

7. Problems of hypnotism

8. Appeal to the patient's automatism

In these chapters Janet goes through the history and details of both hypnosis and suggestion, and some of the connections between them. 'Suggestion' and 'automatisms' are not talked about in those words today, but when you observe the minutiae of modern therapies you can find them. You can suggest a motor movement or action by words or by your own motor movements. You can also suggest discourses to be used but Janet says that motor suggestion is more reliable than the suggesting of word use. Automatisms utilize behaviours which the person already has to change their other behaviours. While these are hidden in most modern therapies, some forms of therapy and hypnosis make a more direct use of these (Erickson, 1980; Erickson, Rossi & Rossi, 1976; Haley, 1973).

Part 3. Psychological economies

9. Treatment by rest

As the name suggests, many treatments involved having the client rest, take a holiday, or relax more. Janet traces the many movements and variations upon such ideas, and the complex criticisms that have been made. In modern therapies these probably still occur but only in the background. There are also some interesting (and very modern) discussions around whether those claiming to be tired or fatigued really are. Janet brings in his own notion here that a person merely has a 'fixed idea' that they are fatigued; in modern terms, that their cognitions are 'faulty' in claiming to be exhausted – it is a language/discursive problem not a bodily exhaustion.

10. Treatment by isolation

Isolation has often been seen as a 'cure' for troubles and Janet reviews the histories of this, including monasteries and retreats, as well as a treatment for 'hysteria' by Charcot and others. Janet then works through some of the possible *component effects* of isolation (a contextual analysis like Chapter 5) and how isolation might be found to help in some circumstances. For some cases of forced isolation, Janet suggested that the person faked being 'cured' in order to be removed from their current bad life situations.

11. Treatment by mental liquidation

In a short but interesting chapter with a strange sounding title (to us), Janet looks at the long-term effects of traumatic events and how people might be rid of these bad effects (of 'mental liquidation'). He brings in much recent work of his own and that of Charcot, Prince, Freud, and Jung (prior to 1919). He is very supportive of the main ideas of Freud except his sexual analyses, especially in a section called 'The exaggerations of psychoanalysis' (p. 640). He also includes a wonderful passage about memory: "*Memory*, like belief, like all psychological phenomena, is an action; essentially, it *is the action of telling a story*" (p. 661, italics in original). This is essentially a contextual analysis conclusion (Guerin, 2016) but 100 years earlier.

Part 4. Psychological acquisitions

12. Education and reeducation

This includes a wide variety of treatments, including the person making movements, bodily exercises, breathing exercises, making eye movements and guiding attention, and acquiring other skills. Some of these share features with what has recently been called variously behavioural activation, behavioural training, and mindfulness methods. Once again, Janet goes through many examples and details the criticisms which have been made.

13. Aesthesiogenic agents

These are treatments in which the person is stimulated or made to produce sensations and include: placing magnets or metals on the person's skin; the person feeling all parts of their skin; hydrotherapy; removing all feelings; and static electricity. Janet is again critical of the way people have talked about these but not of some basic positive results in his examples, which he describes as the person reaching an 'alert state'. He links all these to the previous phenomena he has talked about, such as suggestion and fixed ideas. Some of these are still done (usually with fanciful new stories spun) such as touch healing, Reiki, somatic therapy, and self-touch.

14. Treatment by excitation

These follow from descriptions *12* and *13* and include physical activities and exercise, walking, effort and work, and border on the encouragement of 'willpower'.

15. Psychophysiological methods of treatment

This includes a wide range of treatments, including regular medical procedures, some drugs, and a lot on diet, vegetarianism, and food types. He also discusses the effects of alcohol: "A young man before coming to see me drank ten glasses of brandy 'in order to have sufficient energy to talk', and he was quite free from any disturbances of speech, equilibrium, or memory." (p. 1079). Janet spends longer pointing out the problems with drugs and alcohol, however.

16. Moral guidance

> All the special methods of psychotherapeutics we have been studying under the names of suggestion, moral disinfection, rest, isolation, reeducation, and excitation, were successive outgrowths from the general methods of religious and moralising treatment whose importance was expounded in the first part of this book.
>
> (p. 1112)

Here Janet provides more history of the moral guidance methods and movements.

Common modern psychotherapies and their stated 'treatments' and 'techniques'

The common therapies since the 1950s are not all misguided or wrong, and most do some good. The discourses they have about why they work can usually be disregarded (Chapter 3), but most are getting *some* good outcomes (although some might appear to work because of the time element and other judgement problems to be mentioned in Chapter 9; Lilienfeld, Ritschel, Lynn, Cautin & Latzman, 2014).

So, my advice is to look at what any therapies do and the outcomes of that; and ignore (mostly) what they say, especially anything beyond descriptions of what they observe, and anything abstract or general. Using the same 19 therapies as for Chapter 3, we can now look at what they *report* about their treatments and techniques. In the next chapter I will look more carefully at the *components* of therapies across many different therapies, and why most therapies seem to work at least sometimes for some people. What we will find is that despite the words used, the 19 therapies are all doing similar things with recipients of therapy, and these also match what Janet reported but using different language again.

A more detailed dissection of what therapies do

For the 19 psychotherapies from Chapter 3, the next step was to look at the methods and techniques they report using to achieve their goals (Guerin, 2017). Once again, the procedure I used was the same: examine the writings, videos, and reports of what takes place materially in each of these therapies. What do they say the client and therapists are doing for 50 minutes a week?

Table 4.1 presents the details of the methods reported within these 19 therapies. Please note that I have only listed those most distinct to each therapy. It turns out that most of these therapies use a lot of other techniques, which are the same as others. For example, most therapies get their clients to do some exercises during the week or try something out during the week, but they do not list this as 'behavioural homework', as other do. This is an interesting finding in itself, that methods and techniques are not very unique, despite the marketing.

From this wealth of material, Box 4.2 presents one way of categorizing the sorts of methods and techniques used across these 19 psychotherapies, and Table 4.2 shows how the different component methods from Table 4.1 fit into the categories of Box 4.2. Note how much of this is related to talking and thinking. As will be made clear in Chapter 7, both talking and thinking are really examples of intervening on people's social relationships and discursive communities. If language use and thinking are broken, this is because social relationships are broken.

Table 4.1 The activities reported to be occurring in therapies

Therapy	Activities
Psychoanalysis	Free association Neutrality Empathy Resistance Interpretation Dream interpretation Analysis of transference Analysis of countertransference Core conflictual relationship theme method (wish, real or anticipated responses by others, response of self) Symptom-context method
Jungian Analysis	Using therapeutic relationships to explore Dream analysis Active imagination Creative and artistic explorations Transference and countertransference
Adlerian Therapy	Lifestyle changes (psychotherapy) or within-lifestyle changes (counselling) Therapeutic relationships Family dynamics and constellation Early recollections Lifestyle investigation Dreams Basic mistakes (overgeneralization, impossible goals of security, misperception of life, minimization of self, faulty values and beliefs) Assets Foster social interest Decrease inferiority Changes to lifestyle Change faulty motivation Encouragement Encourage equality Give advice Action techniques (role-playing, empty chair)
Existential Therapy	Find authenticity Therapeutic love Resistance Transference Living and dying Freedom, responsibility, and choice Isolation and loving Meaning and meaninglessness

Therapy	Activities
Person–Centered Therapy	Psychological contact
	Incongruence (client)
	Congruence and genuineness (therapist)
	Unconditional positive regard or acceptance
	Empathy
	Client perceives empathy and acceptance
	Awareness of feelings
	Increase responsibility
	Experience exploration
Gestalt Therapy	Empathy and close relationship
	Enhancing awareness
	Awareness questioning
	Emphasize or exaggerate awareness
	Enhancing awareness through language
	Enhancing awareness through non-verbals
	Enhancing awareness of self and others
	Enhancing awareness of feelings
	Enhancing awareness through self-dialogue
	Enhancing awareness through enactment
	Enhancing awareness through dreams
	Homework
	Enhancing awareness of avoidance
	Integration
	Creativity
	Two-chair technique
Behaviour Therapy	Set goals
	Assess behaviours carefully
	Desensitization
	Relaxation
	Anxiety hierarchies
	Guided imagination
	Imaginal flooding
	In vivo therapies
	Virtual reality therapies
	Live modelling
	Symbolic modelling
	Self-modelling
	Participant modelling
	Covert modelling
	Self-instructions
	Cognitive countering
	Self-monitoring
	Cue-controlled relaxation
	Homework
	Cognitive restructuring
	Eye-movement desensitization
	Positive cognitions or self-statements

Therapy	*Activities*
Acceptance and Commitment Therapy	Acceptance of feelings Recognition of avoidance Cognitive defusion Creative hopelessness
Dialectical Behaviour Therapy	Phone consultations Assess follow-through and commitment Assure safety Experience emotions with less disturbance Increase quality of life through problem solving and changing reactions to problems Attention to social relationships Validation and acceptances strategies Empathy Problem-solving and change Dialectical persuasion from extremes Mindfulness skills Interpersonal skills Distress-tolerance skills
Rational Emotive Behaviour Therapy	Solve immediate problems Identify activating events, irrational beliefs, and consequences Client relationship important Disputing of irrational beliefs Develop more effective philosophy Coping self-statements Cost-benefit analysis Psychoeducational methods Teaching others Problem solving Homework Imagery Role playing Shame-attacking exercises Forceful self-statements Forceful self-dialogue Activity homework Reinforcement and penalties for tasks Skills training
Behavioural Activation Therapy	Build strong relationship Determine treatment goals of activities Modify environments rather than thinking Modifying avoidance activities Functional analysis focusing on broader context Focused activation Task assignment Develop functional routines Attention to experience

Therapy	Activities
Beck Cognitive Therapy	Disrupt cognitive schema from socialization
	Self-monitoring
	Thought sampling
	Collaborative therapeutic relationship
	Guided discovery
	Three-question technique (Socratic: evidence, other interpretations, implications)
	Record automatic thoughts
	Homework
	Not interpretation of automatic thoughts (but experiment or use logical analysis)
	Understand idiosyncratic meaning
	Challenge absolutes
	Reattribution
	Labelling of the distortions
	Decatastrophizing
	Challenge all-or-none thinking
	List advantages and disadvantages
	Cognitive rehearsal
	Behavioural rehearsal
	Social skills training
	Bibliotherapy
Mindfulness-Based Cognitive Therapy	Decenter thoughts
	Defuse thoughts
Schema-Focused Therapy	Focus on childhood development of schema
	Client-therapy relationships important
	Detect schema (abandonment/instability, mistrust/abuse, emotional deprivation, defensiveness/shame, social isolation/shame)
	Imagery or role-playing to activate schema
	Schema dialogue
	Life review of schema (for evidence)
Reality Therapy	Assess doing, thinking, feeling, physiology
	Friendly but firm relationship
	Cycle of wants, direction and doing, evaluation, planning
	Friendly involvement important
	Exploring total behaviour
	Evaluation in sense of assigning values
	Do not accept excuses
	No punishment or criticism
	Don't give up
	Questioning
	Being positive
	Metaphors
	Humour
	Confrontation
	Paradoxical techniques

Therapy	*Activities*
Solution-Focused Therapy	Form collaborative relationship Create expectation of change Complimenting Examine pre-therapy changes Coping questions ("When you get better …"; "How did you do it?") Miracle question ("How would you first know if a miracle cure happened?") Exception-seeking questions Giving the 'message'
Personal Construct Therapy	Understanding the client's story Setting, characterization (antagonists, protagonists, narrator), plot, themes
Narrative Therapy	Listen to stories View stories in new ways Imagine future positive stories Draw maps of the stories Externalize the problem (problem is opponent) Unique outcomes or sparkling moments Alternative narratives Positive narratives Questions about the future Support clients' stories (with family also)
Feminist Therapy	Change not adjustment Self-nurturing and self-esteem Balancing instrumental and relationship strengths Body image Affirming diversity Empowerment and social action Relationship with client most important Cultural analysis Cultural intervention Gender-role analysis and intervention Power analysis and intervention Assertiveness training Reframing and relabelling Demystifying therapy
Other	Hypnosis Pressure method Contextualizing thoughts Suggestion Block critical thoughts Mess up language patterns Challenge from discourse analysis Zen methods Find new audiences for thinking Psychodrama (role reversal, double technique, mirror technique) Fantasy (surplus reality, act fulfilment—changing past events) Future projection Art therapy Dance movement therapy Drama therapy Music therapy

Box 4.2 My categories of what methods or techniques are used in therapies when their jargon is removed

Therapist-Client Social Relationship

>   Building relationships
>   Therapist's style

Modelling, Role-Playing and Homework
Problem-Solving
Dealing with Social Relationships
Dealing with Thinking

>   Getting thoughts
>   Interpreting thoughts
>   Reframing thoughts
>   Challenging/ arguing
>   Blocking thoughts
>   Dealing with 'mistakes/ distortions'
>   Special anxious thoughts
>   Other methods of dealing with thoughts

Dealing with Talking

>   General changes to talking
>   Talking about self
>   Instructions

Looking at (Talking About) Wider Contexts of the Client's Life
Other Method

Table 4.2 One way of reframing the reported activities of therapies into functional groups

Therapist–Client Social Relationship

Building relationships

Analysis of transference (Psychoanalysis)
Analysis of countertransference (Psychoanalysis)
Transference and countertransference (Jung)
Transference (Existential)
Therapeutic relationships (Adler)
Using therapeutic relationships to explore (Jung)
Therapeutic love (Existential)
Close relationship (Gestalt)
Client relationship important (RET)
Build strong relationship (BA)
Client-therapy relationships important (Schema)
Friendly involvement important (Reality)
Relationship with client most important (Feminist)

Psychological contact (PCT)
Congruence and genuineness (therapist) (PCT)
Phone consultations (DBT)
Collaborative therapeutic relationship (CT)
Form collaborative relationship (Solution)

Therapist's style

Empathy (Psychoanalysis)
Empathy (Gestalt)
Empathy (DBT)
Client perceives empathy/ acceptance (PCT)
Understand idiosyncratic meaning (CT)
Understanding the client's story (Personal Construct)
Neutrality (Psychoanalysis)
No punishment or criticism (Reality)
Resistance (Psychoanalysis)
Resistance (Existential)
Friendly but firm relationship (Reality)
Don't accept excuses (Reality)
Confrontation (Reality)
Questioning (Reality)
Encouragement (Adler)
Unconditional positive regard (PCT)
Don't give up (Reality)
Being positive (Reality)
Humour (Reality)
Complimenting (Solution)
Listen to stories (Narrative)

Modelling, Role-Playing and Homework

Action techniques (role-playing, empty chair) (Adler)
Role playing (RET)
Reinforcement and penalties for tasks (RET)
Behavioural rehearsal (CT)
In vivo therapies (Behaviour Therapy)
Virtual reality therapies (Behaviour Therapy)
Homework (Gestalt)
Homework (Behaviour Therapy)
Homework (RET)
Activity homework (RET)
Task assignment (BA)
Homework (CT)
Set goals (Behaviour Therapy)
Assess behaviours carefully (Behaviour Therapy)
Determine treatment goals of activities (BA)
Relaxation (Behaviour Therapy)
Distress-tolerance skills (DBT)
Live modelling (Behaviour Therapy)
Symbolic modelling (Behaviour Therapy)
Self-modelling (Behaviour Therapy)
Participant modelling (Behaviour Therapy)
Psychoeducational methods (RET)

Teaching others (RET)
Skills training (RET)
Develop functional routines (BA)
Problem solving (RET)
Modifying avoidance activities (BA)
Focused activation (BA)
Bibliotherapy (CT)
Change not adjustment (Feminist)

Problem-Solving

Assets (Adler)
Cost-benefit analysis (RET)
List advantages and disadvantages (CT)
Evaluation in sense of assigning values (Reality)
Increase quality of life through problem solving and changing reactions to problems (DBT)
Validation and acceptances strategies (DBT)
Problem-solving and change (DBT)
Solve immediate problems (RET)
Problem-solving and change (Solutions)
Create expectation of change (Solution)
Examine pre-therapy changes (Solution)
Coping questions ("When you get better, …"; "How did you do it?") (Solution)
Miracle question ("How would you first know if a miracle cure happened?") (Solution)
Exception-seeking questions (Solution)

Dealing with Social Relationships

Family dynamics and constellation (Adler)
Foster social interest (Adler)
Interpersonal skills (DBT)
Shame-attacking exercises (RET)
Social skills training (CT)
Assertiveness training (Feminist)
Attention to social relationships (DBT)

Dealing with Thinking

Getting thoughts

Dream interpretation (Psychoanalysis)
Dream analysis (Jung)
Dreams (Adler)
Enhancing awareness through dreams (Gestalt)
Free association (Psychoanalysis)
Active imagination (Jung)
Awareness of feelings (PCT)
Enhancing awareness (Gestalt)
Awareness questioning (Gestalt)
Emphasize or exaggerate awareness (Gestalt)
Enhancing awareness through language (Gestalt)
Enhancing awareness through non-verbals (Gestalt)
Enhancing awareness of self and others (Gestalt)
Enhancing awareness of feelings (Gestalt)
Enhancing awareness through self-dialogue (Gestalt)
Enhancing awareness through enactment (Gestalt)

Enhancing awareness of avoidance (Gestalt)
Forceful self-dialogue (RET)
Identify activating events, irrational beliefs, and consequences (RET)
Imagery (RET)
Guided imagination (Behaviour Therapy)
Recognition of avoidance (ACT)
Thought sampling (CT)
Guided discovery (CT)
Record automatic thoughts (CT)
Detect schema (abandonment/ instability, mistrust/ abuse, emotional deprivation, defensiveness/ shame, social isolation/ shame) (Schema)
Imagery or role-playing to activate schema (Schema)
Pressure method
Hypnosis

Interpreting thoughts

Interpretation of thoughts (Psychoanalysis)

Reframing thoughts

Cognitive countering (Behaviour Therapy)
Cognitive restructuring (Behaviour Therapy)
Eye-movement desensitization (Behaviour Therapy)
Reattribution (CT)
Labelling of the distortions (CT)
Decatastrophizing (CT)
Cognitive rehearsal (CT)
Covert modelling (Behaviour Therapy)
Metaphors (Reality)
Reframing and relabelling (Feminist)
Contextualizing thoughts (BG)

Challenging/ arguing

Dialectical persuasion from extremes (DBT)
Disputing of irrational beliefs (RET)
Develop more effective philosophy (RET)
Three-question technique (Socratic: evidence, other interpretations, implications) (CT)
Challenge absolutes (CT)
Challenge all-or-none thinking (CT)
Challenge from discourse analysis
Paradoxical techniques (Reality)

Blocking thoughts

Decentre thoughts (Mindfulness)
Defuse thoughts (Mindfulness)
Mindfulness skills (DBT)
Block critical thoughts
Mess up language patterns
Zen methods

Dealing with 'mistakes/ distortions'

Basic mistakes (overgeneralization, impossible goals of security, misperception of life, minimization of self, faulty values and beliefs) (Adler)
Cognitive defusion (ACT)
Creative hopelessness (ACT)
Disrupt cognitive schema from socialization (CT)

Special anxious thoughts

Desensitization (Behaviour Therapy)
Anxiety hierarchies (Behaviour Therapy)
Imaginal flooding (Behaviour Therapy)
Experience emotions with less disturbance (DBT)

Other methods of dealing with thoughts

Two-chair technique (Gestalt)
Acceptance of feelings (ACT)
Not interpretation of automatic thoughts but experiment or logical analysis (CT)
Schema dialogue (Schema)
Setting, characterization (antagonists, protagonists, narrator), plot, themes (Personal Construct)

Dealing with Talking

General changes to talking

View stories in new ways (Narrative)
Imagine future positive stories (Narrative)
Draw maps of the stories (Narrative)
Externalize the problem (problem is opponent) (Narrative)
Unique outcomes or sparkling moments (Narrative)
Alternative narratives (Narrative)
Positive narratives (Narrative)
Questions about the future (Narrative)
Support clients' stories (with family also) (Narrative)
New audiences
Psychodrama
Role reversal
Double technique
Mirror technique
Fantasy (surplus reality, act fulfilment—changing past events)
Future projection

Talking about Self

Core conflictual relationship theme method (wish, real or anticipated responses by others, response of self) (Psychoanalysis)
Find authenticity (Existential)
Living and dying (Existential)
Freedom, responsibility, and choice (Existential)
Isolation and loving (Existential)
Meaning and meaninglessness (Existential)
Incongruence (client) (PCT)
Integration (Gestalt)
Focus more on childhood development of schema (Schema)
Life review of schema (for evidence) (Schema)
Body image (Feminist)
Self-nurturing and self-esteem (Feminist)

Instructions

Self-instructions (Behaviour Therapy)
Self-monitoring (Behaviour Therapy)

Cue-controlled relaxation (Behaviour Therapy)
Positive cognitions or self-statements (Behaviour Therapy)
Coping self-statements (RET)
Forceful self-statements (RET)
Self-monitoring (CT)
Suggestion

Looking at Wider Contexts of the Client's Life

Symptom-context method (Psychoanalysis)
Lifestyle changes (psychotherapy) or within-lifestyle changes (counselling) (Adler)
Early recollections (Adler)
Lifestyle investigation (Adler)
Changes to lifestyle (Adler)
Experience exploration (PCT)
Modify environments rather than thinking (BA)
Functional analysis focusing on broader context (BA)
Attention to experience (BA)
Assess doing, thinking, feeling, physiology (Reality)
Cycle of wants, direction and doing, evaluation, planning (Reality)
Exploring total behaviour (Reality)
Balancing instrumental and relationship strengths (Feminist)
Affirming diversity (Feminist)
Empowerment and social action (Feminist)
Cultural analysis (Feminist)
Cultural intervention (Feminist)
Gender-role analysis (Feminist)
Gender-role intervention (Feminist)
Power analysis (Feminist)
Power intervention (Feminist)
Demystifying therapy (Feminist)
Creative and artistic explorations (Jung)
Creativity (Gestalt)

Other

Decrease inferiority (Adler)
Change faulty motivation (Adler)
Encourage equality (Adler)
Give advice (Adler)
Increase responsibility (PCT)
Assess follow-through and commitment (DBT)
Assure safety (DBT)
Giving the 'message' (Solution)
Art therapy
Dance movement therapy
Drama therapy
Music therapy

Having got these methods or techniques extracted, we can now put them into another context. In Chapter 10 we will see three broad ways of supporting people trying to live in restrictive bad life situations (the definition of 'mental health' issues). Level 3 is to try and stop or change the specific behaviours, and Level 2 is caring and supporting the people through their ordeal. Level 1 is actually going out and trying to change those bad life situations directly (Figure 10.1).

With the models of treatment for mental health contextualized from the 19 therapies, we can see that these are almost exclusively Levels 2 and 3. *Very little done by psychotherapists deal directly with solving the bad life situations* (Level 1). The methods either try to change behaviours (Level 1) or to assuage and calm the person and show that someone cares (Level 2). But from within an office, these are both difficult to accomplish (Chapter 2): the first because the person returns to their bad life situations after leaving the office; and the second because this is not 'curing' their bad life situation (even though both are still useful in other ways).

As we will see below, the effects of talking can bring about changes in the person's life situations, but there are special conditions that apply.

To highlight these findings, a further step was conducted. A final analysis of interest is to compare Table 4.2 to a similar list in Table 4.3 made of the activities of *social workers*. These were garnered from a variety of sources listing the skills and activities used by social workers in practice (e.g., Chenoweth & McAuliffe, 2012; Dunk-West, 2013; Schwartz & Goldiamond, 1975; Seabury, Seabury & Garwin, 2011; Trevithick, 2012) but not with the same amount of scope and diligence as was done for the therapies. Just a few comparative points will be made.

First, while a similar emphasis is given to forming a brief stranger/contractual relationship with the clients, there are a lot more activities of the social workers relevant to people from different cultural groups, something very absent in Table 4.2. Second, once the jargon words are removed, there are a lot of convergences in some of the interventions with clients which are listed to those we have found for the psychological therapies in this paper. Hidden in the jargon of Table 4.3 there are many activities by social workers which attempt to change the thoughts and talking of clients: reframing, giving alternative interpretations (verbal), and other counselling skills. There is also the big range of more localized problem-solving interventions as we saw for therapists in Table 4.2. *So, the differences between what therapists and social workers do is much less than many people realize.* It is not the case that social workers just deal with finances, legal aspects, and family conflicts (Level 1) and therapists deal with cognitive processes (Level 3).

The biggest *difference*, however, between social workers and psychotherapists is the much greater engagement by social workers in the lives of the clients, which often equates with what I called Level 1. This is first reflected in the 'gathering details' listing, in which greater attention is paid to varied life contexts such as economic and cultural, and sociological imagination is used (Mills, 1959). The attention to the contexts of the clients' lives is also reflected in the whole section on 'Intervention in client's context', which was noticeably absent in the descriptions of what

Table 4.3 One way of reframing the activities of social workers into functional groups

---

Client Relationship

The ability to create a rapport, connection and a relationship in ways that aid communication/understanding in assessment and intervention processes

Interpersonal skills: an awareness of how we come across and how our own 'use of self' shapes our communication with others

Welcoming skills: the ability to offer a warm greeting/clear introduction

Communication/language skills: articulating an appropriate choice of words and vocabulary when communicating with others

Non-verbal communication skills: taking account of body language in relation to oneself and others

Active listening skills: noting the factual/emotional content of what is being said/not said/use of active responses ('minimum encouragers')

Capacity to engage with others and the task/the ability to be open and changed by the encounter

Emotional attunement skills: responding to the meaning/quality of feelings being expressed/shared

Demonstrating sympathy

Demonstrating empathy

Appropriate use of self-disclosure

Allowing/using silences

Managing professional boundaries and confidentiality requirements

Conveying an appropriate sense of authority/self-confidence and professional accountability in ways that give confidence

Skilled use of touch (e.g., handshake)

Skilled use of humour

Be able to engage and communicate with diverse population and groups of all sizes

Have a knowledge and understanding of human relationships

Active listening

Communicating across culture

Establishing boundaries with clients

Establishing rapport

Inspiring trust

Interacting effectively with diverse clientele

Paraphrasing

Respecting the autonomy of clients

Patience

Positive attitude

Emotional resilience

Gathering details

Observation skills/using the five senses: what we see, hear, smell, taste, and touch, to aid understanding

Memory skills: actively recalling and linking key facts/information

Use of intuition/intuitive reasoning

Information gathering skills: asking good questions/importance of gathering baseline data

Use of open questions

Use of closed questions

Use of *what* questions

Use of *why* questions
Use of circular questions
Use of hypothetical questions
Use of paraphrasing
Use of clarifying
Use of summarizing
Giving feedback thoughtfully
Inviting feedback openly
Use of prompting/probing
Analysing patterns of addiction
Analysing public and social policies
Applying research to social work practices
Assessing family and social factors impacting clients
Assessing the effectiveness of interventions
Conducting research
Continual learning
Analytical, critical thinking
Devising case plans
Documenting case notes
Interviewing
Maintaining confidentiality
Note taking

Interventions with clients

Providing emotional support
Giving advice (cautiously)
Providing information clearly
Providing explanations clearly
Providing encouragement: inspiring /motivating others to take action
Offering affirmation/praise
Providing appropriate reassurance
Breaking 'bad news' sensitively
Social skills training (modelling/demonstrating constructive responses)
Use of reframing
Offering interpretations
Skilfully adapting to need
Use of counselling skills
Containing the anxiety of others
Skills central to self-care/managing our emotional responses
Use of assertiveness skills
Challenging/confrontational skills
Dealing with hostility/aggression
Managing potentially explosive/violent encounters
Improve problem-solving, coping, and development capacities of all people
Provide services to not only support change in the individual but also in his/her environment as well
Calming agitated clients
Caring
Counselling
Customizing treatment plans for addicts
Developing a personal approach to casework and counselling
Instructing
Prioritizing

Problem solving
Providing constructive criticism
Role playing

Interventions in client's context

Skilled use of diplomacy
Skilled use of interventions targeted at wider structural, organizational, and systemic barriers to progress
Organizational/administrative skills: prioritizing, planning, monitoring, and preparing the work at hand
Courtroom skills
Using supervision creatively
Chairing skills: guiding/facilitating contributions from others
Presentation skills: presenting a talk/discussion/public address
Use of telephone skills
Skilled use of mobile phones/text messaging
Recording/form-filling skills
Note taking/minute-taking skills
Use of negotiating skills
Use of contracting skills
Networking skills (formal/informal)
Working in partnership with others in ways that are collaborative, inclusive, unifying, and empowering
Use of mediation skills
Use of advocacy skills
Skilled ability to end a meeting/interview/future contact
Providing help: communicating, emotional warmth, interest, care, concern for others
Providing practical/hands-on assistance
Using persuasion/being directive
Demonstrating leadership skills/initiative/taking decisive action
Advocate for individual clients or the community on identified problems
Serve as a broker by connecting individual with resources
Create and maintain professional helping relationships
Case management
Collaboration
Advising
Advocating for clients
Consulting with other professionals
Making referrals to other service providers
Organizational
Striving to institute social policies which benefit their clientele
Tapping community resources to impact problems
Motivating families to change negative behaviours
Group counselling
Teamwork
Skilled use of social media

psychotherapists do, even if I suggested that some might be done without reporting and some 'off the record'. Social workers have much direct involvement and interventions with people, such as advocacy, negotiation between clients and other people and bureaucracies, and working within the community to assist clients. This presents them with powerful ways to effect change ethically and across the domains of their clients' life worlds, directly as Level 1.

The bigger point perhaps is that if psychological therapists are not doing anything unique by way of their activities, and if they are relying on verbal instructions and verbal shaping using themselves as an audience to guarantee that the client walks away from the clinic with new behaviours which will maintain, then perhaps psychotherapists, psychologists, and psychiatrists *should* be doing a lot more of this direct involvement in a client's life (Level 1). It not only helps with problem solving but will also provide a better platform for creating changes in thinking and talking, which will maintain since the shaping will occur with the real everyday audiences of the client (not the "My therapist said I should not talk like that anymore").

In summary, the main thrusts of almost all the western therapies for goals and activities are to:

- form a working social relationship with a client within a stranger/contractual relationship
- be supportive and caring of them to an extent limited by professional barriers
- work with them to fix the bad life situations they are living in or the legacies of past bad life situations (but mainly by social workers and others)
- solve smaller or more localized conflicts in the client's life, which are amenable within an office
- act as a new audience to train new behaviours and skills where appropriate
- find out their discourses (talking and thinking) around the problems and suffering they have
- attempt to act as a new audience for them to change those thoughts and talking in ways that should be beneficial and reduce the suffering, especially for broader life conflicts

Different therapies focus more or less on different aspects of this, but they all cover much the same ground, or else specialize in only certain types of problems and suffering.

The conclusion for me is that therapists must work in a (usually stranger/contractual) social relationship with the person, and together with other people (1) change the person's bad life situations or the legacies of this, (2) change the person's discourses about their world and themself, (3) and have them behave in some new ways and often the people around them behave in different ways. To do this requires ways of *influencing* or *persuading* the person, but this does not mean hard persuasion or bullying. It means influencing them in ways they are comfortable with, that are ethical, and that will sustain. This often means letting *them* find the ways of 'influencing themselves' as it were, with little therapist involvement, but hopefully they can learn something from the

therapist and use their unconditional support (unconditional except for pay-
ments) in changing what is happening in their lives.

> Although the relationship is voluntary, both hypnosis and therapy
> require persuasion, a selling job, at the beginning of the process. The
> subject or patient must be motivated to cooperate, usually by empha-
> sizing what he [sic] has to gain if he cooperates and what he might lose
> if he does not.
>
> (Haley, 1973, p. 23)

What this implies, also putting this in the context of Janet's work, is that *the
succession of different therapies over the last 50 years has been about new ways to do
these persuasive activities, and not anything more intrinsically different.* Times change
and how people can be influenced and persuaded to change also changes. The
recipients of therapies today are not the same as the recipients of therapies in
the 1950s. Life contexts dramatically change over time, as do societal discourses
and how we talk and converse. *So any differences between older and newer therapies
might be a result of trying the same 'treatment' but having to adapt to a different sort of
population and society.*

The primarily medical people in Janet's time (1925/1919) and in the mid-
1950s (Haley, 1973) *could persuade people using their authority and community pressure*—they could get away with many methods that cannot be used now. In
more recent times, methods have changed, but not because we are getting
closer to 'real' therapies or know better, but *because professional authority has
waned* and the use of legal and governmental control to 'change' people has
increased, including the use of medical drugs as prescriptions by law. Also, with
the waning of professional authority, therapists have been devising new ways of
persuading the people they see to behave and talk (and hence think) differently.
*Most of the newer and third-wave therapies can therefore be seen as just new ways of
persuading different sorts of people to do the same old treatments*, and given that, they
can work. This includes the marketing of therapies, and people might self-select
whichever they will be most persuaded by.

Under these changing historical, societal, social, and cultural contexts, we
would not expect there to be identical ways that therapists could help people at
any time and any place, since all life contexts have changed (for example,
people no longer believing medical and other professionals and having faith in
them as they used to.) Our current social relationships and ways of influencing
people have changed dramatically since the time when 'therapies' started. Here
are some suggestions to follow up:

- *Cognitive behaviour therapies* work using one modern persuasive style of
  bureaucratic, impersonal social relations, avoidance of professional
  authority as that no longer works for many people, and science-looking
  and -sounding discourses with effectiveness and an 'evidence-base' evoked
  as key platforms. Things are set to standards which have publicity that they

work and have been 'proved', even though in reality the details are made up *in situ* for each new person. These marketing efforts are based on very weak ideas of what even makes a 'science' or 'evidence'.

- The *medical model* of social relationship is still very present but social relationships have changed from the 'folksy' local doctor and respected community leader to hospital efficacy and government professionalism, and there is no doubt that the uses of government-ordained powers to have the necessary influence on people (for their own good of course) has increased. Personal medical authority has waned and so we see an increase in administrative and legal rules of authority and power.

- *Third-wave therapies* are likewise dealing with (and are adaptations to) new forms of social relationships in our societies. They have not discovered new truths about doing therapies but have adapted to the failing of old ways to persuade people (such as those in Janet). Some are called post-modernist because it is clear they are adaptations to *new forms of social relationships*, and so language, word plays, and less formalized methods are used (Anderson, 1997). This is not because they have been proved efficacious for everyone, but because there is a new audience who no longer go along with older forms of building social relationships (such as faith in professionals to do the right thing). Many take on an informal and 'I am your friend and buddy' approach to accomplish the same goals, which go back to Janet and beyond.

- Finally, *looking ahead to the future*, the current 'younger' generations are growing up in a world which is different again. Serious social relationships and becoming 'buddies' with adults is extremely tenuous and lacking in trust for anything concrete (with good reason). This suggests a further tightening will occur of being forced by law for compliance (which is the wrong strategy of course, but 'prodromal' plans for 'mental health' are already beginning to do this). Following further the 'post-modern' movements, any form of 'authenticity' or marketing will also not work to engage social relationships let alone allow cooperative progress, as younger generations are no longer fooled by these and have a much improved healthy cynicism of how the current world is played out by governments, corporations, and people (e.g., Katz, Ogilvie, Shaw & Woodhead, 2021). Social media and the internet will also mean that people thinking about therapy will be well ahead in knowing what is really going on, or else influenced first by 'social media influencers' (Baker & Rojek, 2020). Therapists are really going to have to work collaboratively and perhaps take a step back to become a minor party in any therapeutic relationship (this book is already suggesting that a single therapist per client model is not working).

Conclusions

So the point I take from the analyses of this chapter and the last are that most therapies are talking therapies and all have similar reported goals and methods wrapped up in very different discourses, explanations and marketing. This has been the case for some time (Janet, 1925/1919). But this does not mean that they do not do some good. Most are aimed at supporting the person through their troubles to different degrees, and all attempt to change what a person is doing in their bad life situations almost exclusively by persuading them in very different ways, through the use of words.

'Improvements' in therapies, and new therapies, are characterized mainly by finding a new discourse to wrap what they do in descriptions and explanations, and these are successively being reshaped towards changes in social relationships, which have occurred in societies with new societal rules, discourses, and practices. The next generations will shape new sets of theories and discourses, because they will both listen and be persuaded to talk differently in different and new ways, but the practices will basically remain the same as Janet (e. g., Katz, Ogilvie, Shaw & Woodhead, 2021).

Of most concern is that when the problems involved are seen as being shaped by a person's contexts, societal economic, social relationship, etc., then psychotherapies do very little to directly address this (Level 1). Social work does a lot more. I will come back to this in later chapters, as this needs to be addressed more than finding new ways to talk to people in therapy.

References

Addiss, S. (2008). *Zen sourcebook: Traditional documents from China, Korea and Japan*. Indianapolis, IN: Hackett.

Anderson, H. (1997). *Conversation, language, and possibilities: A postmodern approach to therapy*. NY: Basic Books.

Baker, S. A., & Rojek, C. (2020). *Lifestyle gurus: Constructing authority and influence online*. London: Polity.

Chenoweth, L., & McAuliffe, D. (2012). *The road to social work & human service practice*. Melbourne: Cengage Learning.

Dunk-West, P. (2013). *How to be a social worker: A critical guide for students*. NY: Palgrave Macmillan.

Erickson, M. H. (1980). *Innovative hypnotherapy. The collected papers of Milton H. Erickson on hypnosis*, Vol. 4. NY: Irvington Publishers.

Erickson, M. H., Rossi, E. L., and Rossi, S. I. (1976). *Hypnotic realities: The induction of clinical hypnosis and forms of indirect suggestion*. NY: Irvington.

Fairbank, J. K. (1957). *Chinese thought and institutions*. Chicago: University of Chicago Press.

Guerin, B. (2016). *How to rethink human behavior: A practical guide to social contextual analysis*. London: Routledge.

Guerin, B. (2017). Deconstructing psychological therapies as activities in context: What are the goals and what do therapists actually do? *Revista Perspectivas em Análise do Comportamento, 8*, 97–119.

Hadot, P. (1995). *Philosophy as a way of life: Spiritual exercises from Socrates to Foucault*. London: Blackwell.

Haley, J. (1973). *Uncommon therapy: The psychiatric techniques of Milton H. Erickson, M. D.* New York: Norton.

Janet, P. (1924). *Principles of psychotherapy*. NY: Macmillan.

Janet, P. (1925/1919). *Psychological healing: A historical and clinical study.* London: George Allen & Unwin.

Katz, R., Ogilvie, S., Shaw, J., & Woodhead, L. (2021). *Gen Z, explained: The art of living in a digital age.* Chicago: University of Chicago Press.

Lilienfeld, S. O., Ritschel, L. A., Lynn, S. J., Cautin, R. L. & Latzman, R. D. (2014). Why ineffective psychotherapies appear to work: A taxonomy of causes of spurious therapeutic effectiveness. *Perspectives on Psychological Science, 9,* 355–387.

Mills, C. W. (1959). *The sociological imagination.* Oxford: Oxford University Press.

Schwartz, A., & Goldiamond, I. (1975). *Social casework: A behavioral approach.* NY: Columbia University Press.

Seabury, B. A., Seabury, B. H., & Garwin, C. D. (2011). *Foundations of interpersonal practice in social work: Promoting competence in generalist practice.* NY: Sage.

Trevithick, P. (2012) *Social work skills & knowledge: A practice handbook* (3rd Ed.). London: Open University Press.

5 How do therapists respond?

Implicit and explicit social relationships of therapies

Having looked in more detail at the reported goals and the broad methods of therapies, we now 'deconstruct' the different therapies into more detailed 'components'. One problem we confront is that therapists of different sorts have worked with people for over a century, but how those therapies have worked is not as clear cut (Guerin, 2020). The methods they use might truly be beneficial, but if one reads the writing of therapists with a critical discursive approach, so much of it is metaphor and storytelling (Chapters 1, 3 and 4). As was pointed out earlier, we should not take the theories of therapists themselves as being authentic or privileged in any sense. We must keep separate what therapists say, what they say they do, and what they are observed to do.

We should therefore be careful in attributing change to what we can talk about, and the therapists' theories and claims for why they have been successful:

- because the bad life situations might change independently of any 'therapy' or 'helping' just because life events have changed (Chapter 9)
- because some independent change brought the person to therapy in the first place and that might also be what actually helped them (Guerin, 2005)
- because there are life situations and changes which we *cannot* put into words (Guerin, 2020)
- because the metaphors and stories spun around therapies might be placating to hear, but that does not mean the therapist has pinpointed the change components (Lilienfeld, Ritschel, Lynn, Cautin & Latzman, 2014).

In the following, I do *not* wish to give an exhaustive study of all therapies and forms of healing. My goal is to get the reader thinking about what is actually done when someone 'gives therapy' to another person, by pointing out and illustrating many *implicit components* which are usually ignored in any discourses and 'evidence base'. I want to put this in different contexts to provide more flexible thinking around the issues involved, rather than give one supposedly final account.

DOI: 10.4324/9781003300571-6

Two components of therapy that might be efficacious, but which have nothing to do with the therapy per se

Two important considerations of what makes therapies work will be given here briefly but more will be developed in Chapter 9.

Time

First, people's life situations change over time in most cases, so a lot of the change in therapy we observe might be nothing to do with the therapy itself. This would be especially true for younger people who are still developing and changing, and their life contexts with them, and for anyone in therapy for longer than six months. Over six months or so in therapy, and we would expect changes to have taken place in people's lives, especially younger people. In fact, if no change, during six months of therapy, has taken place this can tell us something about their life situations as well.

What gets you to seek help or therapy

A second point is that for those who go to some sort of designated 'therapist', 'helper' or 'healer', we must also look closely at the contexts for 'What got them to go at all?' (Guerin, 2005). In many cases, whatever got them to go for help in the first place, whether a nagging partner, a new discourse they discovered, or a slight change in their context, could also be the contextual change which brings about any behaviour change that gets attributed to the therapy (Lilienfeld, Ritschel, Lynn, Cautin & Latzman, 2014). Sometimes people do not seek 'help' until it seems that things are starting to get better already; if things remain really bad, then they do not seek help.

General components of most 'therapies' which might lead to beneficial changes

Below are some simple analyses of the more detailed contexts for therapy and what components might be working. My problem is not so much the lack of evidence of outcomes, but that currently most of the therapies do not *analyse* what might be affecting a person's life world when they do these activities, especially how these activities might improve their bad situations. They still assume that (1) the change is made 'within' the person and (2) *their named activity* is what led to this change (such as *tree-hugging* therapy, Guerin, 2020, or '*Watching the stars*' therapy, see below). Even the 'scientific' evidence is focused only on these points, especially that the outcomes have been brought about by the *therapist-named* components. In fact, every one of these therapies I have seen involves a huge number of changes to the person's life contexts, and in many cases I really doubt that the *named* activity (the marketing) is what is bringing about these therapeutic changes, or at least not that alone.

Box 5.1 explores *what else might be bringing about changes in therapies* other than what is named or theorized by the therapists and researchers (which we saw in Chapters 3 and 4). Box 5.1 gives some examples which occur in some form in almost all types of therapies, in addition to the named or marketed methods and techniques (Guerin, 2017).

Box 5.1 Events occurring in most therapies, in addition to the named or marketed methods and techniques, and which might be bringing about any changes found.

- during the time of therapy, independent changes have occurred in the person's life (I mentioned this just above); the longer the therapy, the more likely that this occurs
- some change has already led the person to carry out, in addition to the named or marketed methods and techniques, this therapy *at all*, and *how that was done* might be the strongest force in itself (I mentioned this just above, and see Guerin, 2005)
- getting out of the house for therapy, gets the person out of their bad situations for a while; removes the person from their normal contexts in which their common bad situations take place; provides escape by getting out of the physical settings and what they shape
- doing some new activity
- 'researching' therapies online or through books leads to other discoveries of context
- more engagement in life in a general sense by talking to someone, albeit in an office
- moving your behaviour away from language-based conflicts
- joining in social groups to change their world in some new way, entertainments of all sorts, music, concerts, travel, crafts, performance, arts, study, reading, alterative religions, and general activities like walking, sports or yoga
- unblock alternatives you could not do in the bad situation; give new alternatives for behaviour and thinking
- contact with new people – I have frequently heard from people with firsthand experience that making *'social connections'* was vitally important in helping them through their bad situations (whether this is the therapist or others)
- new life possibilities coming from meeting new people (resource-social relationship pathways)
- provides possible new social relationships or helps break out of the old ones
- provision of new stories and other discourses for their normal audiences about this new activity

- useful new discourses gained from listening to those involved in the new activity (could be advice, alternative possibilities, stories about others in similar bad situations, Janet's 'suggestions')
- exploration of alternative discourses and thoughts
- various therapeutic experiences might also provide many alternative self-identity discourses to tell people back in the original bad life context, and this will change how those people then interact
- provide escape from the monitoring and evaluation by others
- provide opportunities for secrecy when back in the bad situation

So, I am not arguing that only these activities have effects, just that the named or marketed therapeutic activities ('cognitive reframing', 'mindfulness', 'dream analysis') are not what necessarily lead to any changes. The problem is that with so many potential components occurring in every therapy, being successful for one person or for one bad situation does not mean it will work for others. Only observations in context will tell us. Similar events can take place in other life activities as well (Ansdell, 2014; DeNora, 2011, 2015; Moyle, 1986).

I have previously given a fictitious example of these potential components through *tree-hugging* therapy (Guerin, 2020). Let me give another example to make the points clear and call it '*Watching the stars*' therapy (the celestial bodies, not celebrity people; although it could be either). Please note that this is not mocking alternative theories; in fact, it is showing how there can still be useful effects, even if the 'named activity' and marketing is *not* what is shaping any effective changes. I believe many of these alternative therapies are often having good effects for people but not necessarily changing their 'mental health' behaviours directly, and that any changes are not because of the 'named activity'. The main point for the reader is that if the *Tree-hugging* therapy or the '*Watching the stars*' therapy were found to be successful it would *not* be because of the actual tree-hugging or watching of stars.

Imagine this scenario: for those living in bad and restrictive situations who have developed some of the 'mental health' behaviours (Chapter 9) or suffer from the legacies of such bad life situations (Chapter 10), we '*somehow*' (my earlier point) manage to get them to agree to do *Watching the stars* therapy. This involves paying some money to a 'therapist', who one night a week picks up the 'clients' in a little bus and drives them away from the city lights. The drive is about two hours away, but they have warm coffee and tea available, and some snacks. They might do this five to six times together. Once out in the countryside, they go to the top of a little hill together with a short walk. Blankets and fold-up chairs are provided and everyone (maybe ten people maximum?) sits down and consumes the drinks and snacks together.

Once settled, and when it is dark (different procedures will apply when cloudy or rainy), everyone moves a little away from each other and sits or lies down on individual blankets or fold-up chairs. They then spend about 60 or more minutes watching the stars without talking or contact, but still in the presence of each other. After this, they get back together but are not asked about what they saw or thought about. They just talk about whatever they wish, and people listen to them. Usually they tell stories to each other, only sometimes about the stars, sometimes about their lives, and sometimes just swap funny or entertaining stories. There is no demand to answer any questions or talk about their bad life situations, but this can be done if two of the people agree. No one should be trying to fix the other people.

Table 5.1 shows some of the possible components from Box 5.1 of this new *Watching the stars* therapy.

The point from here is that *many of these components also occur during mainstream psychotherapy sessions* (PTh), although many are explicitly excluded (like meeting with your therapist out of the office or lying down on the floor). Learning new discourses is usually possible in mainstream therapies, even though the discourses might be limited to theories, abstract concepts and rules to be followed, and a single therapist. On the other hand, most therapies *ask* an awful lot of questions and have this as a hidden but permanent demand on the client (more on this later in this chapter).

Many of the weirder-looking therapies and methods of 'healing' discussed by Janet (1925/1919; Box 4.1) can also be analysed into the types of outcomes in Box 5.1. Some of Janet's category 'Miraculous healings', for example, can be analysed in these terms and more. Once again, they might have some positive effects for the clients, but not because of the 'named' explanation for the outcome or the therapist's theoretical reasons and marketing (they are not miracles but due to these other component events).

Ways of responding in therapies as important components

Since most modern therapies (such as the 19 given previously) consist primarily of talking, it is also worthwhile looking more closely at how therapists conduct their conversations. How a therapist responds to and talks with their recipients is yet another *component* event, but one which has had some discussion already in the literature, especially starting with Carl Rogers and forms of 'non-directive' therapy. But there is a lot more hidden here (Guerin, Ball & Ritchie, 2021),

Commonly in current therapies, *a lot of questions are asked*, at least at the beginning of therapy. These typically focus on the person's history, presenting issues, a little context but not in great detail, and often some procedural matters. Such questions clearly depend on whether the person is talking to a clinical psychologist, psychiatrist, social worker, counsellor, psychotherapist, etc. Some ask more about medical and physical context, few ask about social and economic context. Those who still do DSM diagnoses (whether willingly or not), usually focus questions on the minimum needed to reach a diagnosis, and often not much more is asked or said after that about the clients' life contexts.

Table 5.1 Some of the possible component events of this new *Watching the stars* therapy

Some incidental outcomes of the therapeutic set-up	Examples from *Watching the stars* therapy. Those which probably occur in most mainstream psychotherapies have 'PTh' written
Time	This might occur over a few months and independent changes might occur for people in their lives during this time PTh
Some change has already led the person to agree to carry this out *at all*, and *how that was done* might be the strongest force for change in itself (Guerin, 2005)	What was it that got the person to agree to go to *Watching the stars* therapy? Whatever that was, might be the event that shaped the change PTh
Getting out of the house, gets you out of the bad situations for a while; removing the person from their normal contexts in which their common bad situations take place; provide escape by getting out of the physical settings and what they shape	Whatever bad life situation the person is in, *Watching the stars* therapy gets them away from that for a time PTh
Doing some new activities	The person gets to do some new behaviours, even including walking, sitting on a bus, using a new form of public transport, sitting or lying down, communal meal, star gazing, with no demands
More engagement in life in a general sense	Out of the house the person is engaging in life itself in new ways
Unblock alternatives you could not do in the bad situation; give new alternatives for behaviour and thinking	Often alternative activities or strategies are blocked by others in the bad life situations, so going out and doing new activities without those people can allow some of those previously punished or blocked to appear and be shaped PTh
Joining in social groups to change their world in some new way, entertainments of all sorts, music, concerts, travel, crafts, performance, arts, study, reading, alternative religions, and general activities like walking, sports or yoga	They not only meet new people but learn from those people about other life activities which they could try, and they are meeting similar people to themselves
Move your behaviour away from language-based conflicts	Many of the bad life situations involve words and conflict of words, so this takes them away from that into a space with nice words and no demand that words be used, they can just watch stars silently if they wish
Provides contact with new people; I have frequently heard from people with firsthand experience that making 'social connections' was vitally important in helping them through their bad situations	They can meet new people who are similar in some ways, but who do not know of anyone else's bad life situation; the people in this therapy are probably similar in many ways

New life possibilities coming from meeting new people (resource-social relationship pathways)	Meeting new people can lead to other events and social relationships, even outside of this therapy
Can assist to break out of the old social relationships	Meeting new people on the trip can also help replacing dependence on those in the bad life situations, and start afresh, more than your single therapist PTh
Provision of new stories and other discourses for their normal audiences about this new activity	Exposure to a new range of discourses from new people with diverse backgrounds; more than your single therapist PTh
Useful new discourses gained from listening to those involved in the new activity (could be advice, alternative possibilities, stories about others in similar bad situations)	They can hear new discourses related to their own bad life situations; the *Watching the stars* therapy can also give a bigger or new perspective on the discourses a person has about their life events; more than your single therapist PTh
Shape alternative discourses and thoughts	They can begin thinking or saying discourses which previously have been punished in their bad life situations; which had been shaped to be thought only (with anxiety) or dissociated and dissociachotic (Ball & Picot, 2021) PTh
Various therapeutic experiences might also provide many alternative self-identity discourses to tell to people back in the original bad life context, and this will change how those people then interact	Supports more positive self-discourses, which might carry back to the bad situations at the end of the day PTh
Provide escape from the monitoring and evaluation by others	A period away from the bad life situations and the monitoring, questioning and evaluation by others
Provide opportunities for secrecy when back in bad situation, and have unique experiences	Provides some stories and experiences which can remain secret when back in bad life situations, which can support alternative self-discourses and maintain them against the bad life situations PTh

As I will argue, for those coming to therapy in crisis, asking questions is not a good way to respond to them.

As we saw in Chapters 3 and 4, most of the psychotherapies have similar goals and outcomes, but only a few of the psychotherapies have concentrated on *how to respond* (e.g., Rogers, 1951). Most others focus on the content of what needs to be found out and the questions to be asked.

But both the content and the 'How should we respond to clients?' clearly depend upon all the contexts of therapy. As mentioned in Chapter 2, most therapies are between strangers and done for money, with strong confidentiality (even from the client's family), and with little or no social influence from the therapist to force clients to do anything in particular (the client can get up and leave if they wish, unless under there are legal orders through a psychiatrist). The money payment can also have hidden implications that some 'improvement' is expected from the therapy, and that failure to improve can be attributed to the other person's fault.

So, a lot of the 'techniques' or responding which have grown over the last decades are as much about these *tenuous social contexts* and *persuasion* than anything useful for the client. Here is an early version (based on Pierre Janet's work) which is very different from most of the 'techniques' today in which finding a DSM category is paramount, but similar methods are being instigated once again as faith in the current approaches diminishes:

> ... the simple rules for the conduct of any clinical interview, whether medical or sociological, are as follows:
>
> 1 Give your whole attention to the person interviewed, and make it evident that you are doing so.
> 2 Listen—don't talk.
> 3 Never argue, never give advice.
> 4 Listen to:
> 5 What he [sic] wants to say.
> 6 What he does not want to say.
> 7 What he cannot say without help.
> 8 As you listen, plot out tentatively and for subsequent correction the pattern that is being set before you. To test this, occasionally summarize what has been said and present it for comment. Always do this with caution—that is, abbreviate and clarify but do not add or "twist".
> 9 Remember that everything said must be considered a personal confidence and not divulged to anyone. (This does not prevent discussion of a situation between professional colleagues. Nor does it prevent some form of public report when due precaution has been taken.)
>
> (Mayo, 1948, p. 23)

The point being made is that how therapists interact with or respond to recipients are not just an innocent gleaning of information—*they are integral components of the social context for therapy and much of the success or not might be attributed to this.*

The top half of Box 5.2 gives some contemporary and commonly taught ways to interact with and respond to clients (we will come to the bottom half later – alternative therapeutic responses to clients). The emphasis is on getting them to talk and say how they feel, and also with questions to find about their history and the behaviours they are experiencing. A client who is just silent is not seen in a positive way usually. A client who cries or shows other emotions is okay, but they are then encouraged to *talk* about that emotion. As said earlier, the goal is usually to get enough verbal information from the client to assist in fixing their problem, but this usually means giving them words and discourses to talk about their problem, not to actually change their bad life situations more directly.

Box 5.2 How do therapists respond to help?

Common contemporary therapeutic responses to clients

"How do you feel?"
Reflect back what the client said
Talk in ways to show respect
Try and respond positively and optimistically if possible
Talk in ways to encourage them to say more
Talk in ways to encourage them to give more detail or context
Talk in ways to show that you have had similar experiences to theirs
Talk in ways to fix the person's problems
Give advice
Nodding or saying "Hmm", "Yes", etc.

Alternative therapeutic responses to clients

Not ask questions (especially in crises) as this can be punishing
Hug and touch
Joking
Just listening and say little ('Just Listening')
Reflect how what the client said made you feel ('Emotional CPR')
Just be there without doing or trying anything specific
Do non-language things (sing, rhythms, draw, sketch in sand)
Story telling

The responses in the bottom part of Box 5.2 come mostly from more recent therapies, which are non-pathologizing (non-medical models) and non-diagnostic (cf. Guerin, Ball & Ritchie, 2021). Many of these responses in the bottom half of Box 5.2 are already known from other sources of therapy and relationship building, at least as components, such as Open Dialogue and similar methods (Bergström, Seikkula, Alakare, Mäki, Köngas-Saviaro, Taskila, Tolvanen & Aaltonen, 2018; Parker, Schnackenberg & Hopfenbeck, 2021; Razzaque, 2019; Seikkula, 2020), ethnography (Bohannan & van der Elst, 1998; Cubellis, 2020; Goulet, 1998), and Indigenous listening (Chamberlain, Gee, Gartland, et al., 2020). Some were propounded by Janet (in the earlier Mayo quote).

In most cases in the bottom half, the immediate goal is not to 'fix the person', unlike the 19 psychotherapies given in previous chapters. This is especially important when a person is in crisis, since making demands is not the best form of interaction, and in these contexts, asking a lot of questions will be seen as making demands. This will lead to shutting down of any interaction and social relationships (dissociachotic, Ball & Picot, 2021). Even getting them to put their emotions into words will be seen as demanding, from the context of their bad life situations—even more so when the emotions are there precisely because there are not words for what the person is experiencing (Guerin, 2020). So, they should experience the emotion but not try to put it into words.

Other therapies add more 'natural' human interaction (as occurs in *Watching the stars* therapy), such as joking and touching where appropriate. Others focus on 'methods' best seen in 'Just Listening', in which there is no attempt to 'fix' the person, but simply to listen to them tell their own story. Others just do whatever activities the person wants to do. Others engage the person (if they wish) in non-language-based activities such as singing, making rhythms, drawing, sketching in sand, dancing, art, music. This is very different to most current 'art therapies' and 'music therapies', which use these activities *to get the person to talk* about their history and experiences (Guerin, 2019; Killick, 2017), or to use words (and jargon often) to *interpret* these activities.

Finally, the methods called 'Emotional CPR' are an interesting mixture (Browning & Waite, 2010; Myers, Collins-Pisano, Ferron, & Fortuna, 2021). With this you do not reflect back to the client what they have told you, as many forms of counselling and therapy teach. Instead, the idea is to (genuinely) let the person know *how what they said has affected you*. For example, if someone said, "*I feel like I am useless and my life is going nowhere*", you do *not* respond with, "*What I hear is that you feel your life is a waste of time and you can do nothing useful*". Instead, you might respond with, "*You know, that makes me sad when I hear you say that*". Or, "I feel happy hearing that because I used to talk that way but no longer do, so there is hope". What is said depends upon the authentic way you felt after hearing the client speak. You might also possibly say, "*I laughed inside when you said that, because it reminded me of Marvin the Paranoid Android*".

What is interesting in the E-CPR (Emotional CPR) approach is that when someone is in crisis, they probably have very little or no effect in their worlds (Chapter 9). No one in their social relationships (and maybe these are few) listens to them or pays attention, and no one does anything the person might ask (or they would have changed the situation long before). Whatever they might say by way of bonding or getting people to do things, does not work. It is like their language is broken. While reflecting back to such a client what they tell you lets them know you are listening, *there is no indication that what they say has an effect on the therapist at all*. Reflecting back can sometimes even sound like a parrot and can be programmed on computers, as we know.

However, I believe that E-CPR's benefit, no matter what is said (even about Marvin), is powerful *precisely because* the person knows that what they said actually had an effect in the world; someone was affected by something they said or did. This goes against most therapeutic methods of how therapists should interact with their clients (top of Box 5.2), in that (1) you talk about yourself, and (2) honestly say how you were affected. But in the context of the client's contexts, this can be extremely important to them (see more in Guerin, Ball & Ritchie, 2021). I will come back to alternative ways to conduct 'therapy' in later chapters.

References

Ansdell, G. (2014). *How music helps in music therapy and everyday life.* London: Routledge.

Ball, M., & Picot, S. (2021). Seeing the non-psychosis that we share. *Journal of Humanistic Psychology*, 61, 1–8.

Bergström, T., Seikkula, J., Alakare, B., Mäki, P., Köngas-Saviaro, P., Taskila, J. J., Tolvanen, A., & Aaltonen, J. (2018). The family-oriented open dialogue approach in the treatment of first-episode psychosis: Nineteen-year outcomes. *Psychiatry Research*, 270, 168–175.

Bohannan, P. & van der Elst, D. (1998). *Asking and listening: Ethnography as personal adaptation.* Long Grove, IL: Waveland Press.

Browning, S., & Waite, R. (2010). The gift of listening: JUST listening strategies. *Nursing Forum*, 45, 150–158.

Chamberlain, C., Gee, G., Gartland, D., Mensah, F. K., Mares, S., Clark, Y., Ralph, N., Atkinson, C., Hirvonen, T., McLachlan, H., Edwards, T., Herman, H., Brown, S. J., & Nicholson, J. M. (2020). Community perspectives of complex trauma assessment for Aboriginal parents: "It's important, but *how* these discussions are held is critical". *Frontiers in Psychology*, 11, 1–17.

Cubellis, L. (2020). Sympathetic care. *Cultural Anthropology*, 35, 14–22.

DeNora, T. (2011). *Music-in-action: Selected essays in sonic ecology.* Burlington, VT: Ashgate.

DeNora, T. (2015). *Music asylums: Wellbeing through music in everyday life.* London: Routledge.

Goulet, J-G. A. (1998). *Ways of knowing: Experience, knowledge, and power among the Dene Tha.* Lincoln: University of Nebraska Press.

Guerin, B. (2005). *Handbook of interventions for changing people and communities.* Reno, Nevada: Context Press.

Guerin, B. (2017). Deconstructing psychological therapies as activities in context: What are the goals and what do therapists actually do? *Revista Perspectivas em Análise do Comportamento*, 8, 97–119.

Guerin, B. (2019). Contextualizing music to enhance music therapy. *Revista Perspectivas em Análise Comportamento*, 10, 222–242.

Guerin, B. (2020). *Turning mental health into social action.* London: Routledge.

Guerin, B., Ball, M., & Ritchie, R. (2021). *Therapy in the absence of psychopathology and neoliberalism.* University of South Australia: Unpublished paper.

Janet, P. (1925/1919). *Psychological healing: A historical and clinical study.* London: George Allen & Unwin.

Killick, K. (Ed.). (2017). *Art therapy for psychosis: Theory and practice.* London: Routledge.

Lilienfeld, S. O., Ritschel, L. A., Lynn, S. J., Cautin, R. L. & Latzman, R. D. (2014). Why ineffective psychotherapies appear to work: A taxonomy of causes of spurious therapeutic effectiveness. *Perspectives on Psychological Science*, 9, 355–387.

Mayo, E. (1948). *Some notes on the psychology of Pierre Janet.* Cambridge, MA: Harvard University Press.

Moyle, R. M. (1986). *Alyawarra music: Songs and society in a central Australian community.* Canberra: Australian Institute of Aboriginal Studies.

Myers, A. L., Collins-Pisano, C., Ferron, J. C., & Fortuna, K. L. (2021). Feasibility and preliminary effectiveness of a peer-developed and virtually delivered community mental health training program (Emotional CPR): Pre-Post study. *Journal of Participatory Medicine*, 13, 1–11.

Parker, I., Schnackenberg, J., & Hopfenbeck, M. (Eds.). (2021). *The practical handbook of hearing voices: Therapeutic and creative approaches.* London: PCCS Books.

Razzaque, R. (2019). *Dialogical psychiatry: A handbook for the teaching & practice of Open Dialogue.* London: Omni House Press.

Rogers, C. R. (1951). *Client-centered therapy.* Cambridge, MA: The Riverside Press.

Seikkula, J. (2020). From research on dialogical practice to dialogical research: Open Dialogue is based on a continuous scientific analysis. *Systemic Research in Individual, Couple, and Family Therapy and Counseling*, 7, 143–164.

Part 2

A new approach to stop pathologizing and exoticizing 'mental health'

6 What is different with social contextual analyses?

In this chapter and the next I will do a little introduction to social contextual analysis (SCA), but I will do this in a more practical way involving therapy about how to observe and analyse what people are doing, and mainly just for dealing with 'mental health' behaviours. For a broader and more detailed introduction you can see the full references (Guerin, 2016a, 2016b, 2017, 2020a, 2020b, 2020c).

Social contextual analysis is not a brand-new way to understand why people do what they do, including why people do the 'mental health' behaviours we observe. It is based on some earlier research in psychology (especially that of J. J. Gibson and behaviour analysis) but draws mostly on the contextual analyses of all the social sciences (Guerin, 2020a, 2020b).

Social contextual models of behaviour

The main starting point for social contextual analysis is that human behaviours (doing, talking, thinking, feeling) do not *originate* from internal states or events (Chapter 1). Such explanations in terms of internal brain processes, abstract cognitive processes, or abstract 'internal states' (feelings, personality, mind, etc.) have been the standard way psychology has historically 'explained' human behaviour (see Figures 1.1, 1.2 and 1.3).

The problem is that these are all arbitrary and abstract, and we have no way of even observing these. This is not saying, please note, that our internal physiology and brain stuff are not involved or important in our behaviours—they are indeed. But how we do things, see things, feel things, say things, and think things, do not *originate* or *start* inside us.

Now, the typical way of opposing such internal origins of behaviour in the history of psychology and philosophy has been to move to an extreme or narrow form of explaining everything we do by an immediate 'stimulus' in the environment: for each response there must be a stimulus object which triggered or originated that response. If we can just find that 'stimulus' we can explain the behaviour. But wrong again!

This is obviously too simple to be true, and there are two mistakes made in this. First, a mistake in assuming there must be one stimulus per one response.

DOI: 10.4324/9781003300571-8

We humans are far too nuanced for that! The second mistake is in treating the 'stimulus' only as an 'object' in the physical environment. Instead, our human 'environments' must include *all* the worlds in which we actively engage, and this includes our social, societal, cultural, discursive, economic, and opportunity worlds, not just the chairs and tables around us. These all shape our behaviours.

That is why I use the word 'context' instead of 'environment', to remind us that we are looking at all the bits of how we engage with and are shaped by all these worlds. This also means, in passing, that to understand human behaviour you need a good knowledge of sociology, social anthropology, sociolinguistics, etc. You need to analyse *all* these contexts to figure out (analyse) why people do what they do. In the next section of this book, I am going to apply this to 'mental health' and to therapy.

The final introductory point concerns the *social* in 'social contextual analysis'. This is added because other people and society are enmeshed in *everything* we do as humans, even when it looks superficially like we are 'acting alone'. We will see below that this even applies to what is called 'thinking' and 'consciousness'. As many in the social sciences have been saying for over a century, the idea of an individual self-contained and self-controlling human, originating their own independent decisions inside their heads, is a total myth (Guerin, 2001, 2016a). We are all idiosyncratic, to be sure, but we cannot be independent of the worlds in which we engage. And we are idiosyncratic *because* we are shaped by idiosyncratic worlds.

Most of psychology and psychiatry therefore assume (wrongly) that we are individuals and we 'decide' and 'choose' for 'ourselves (somewhere inside us). To cover some obvious social influences, they then claim that these 'individual' humans have social *factors* or social *determinants* acting on them, as if there was a socially free 'inner' individual who then gets bombarded by social factors! This whole model and way of thinking is misguided but that is the essence of cognitive theory, amongst many others. Our 'inner' cognitive processes are socially free, even if we 'process' social information. (Tip: the words 'factors' and 'determinants' are a red flag for me; they warn me that the way humans are shaped *in their very construction* by 'the social' has not been appreciated and appropriately understood.)

Our (so-called) 'inner' workings are shaped in the very first place (since birth) by our social, societal, and cultural worlds; our 'self' is a verbal construction shaped by external social and societal worlds, a way of talking about ourselves *with which we engage with our social worlds* (Guerin, 2020b). When we commonly talk about our 'inner' self or someone working out their 'internal problems', this is a shorthand for talking about their ways of talking and writing, their discourses, and these are constructed and being reshaped by other people.

Resource–social relationship pathways are our lives

So, the 'social' in social contextual analysis is there to remind you (and me) that there is no socially independent human person somewhere 'inside' us.

Everything we do and we are, has been shaped by our social worlds, since everything we get from the non-social world comes through other people and societal structures: nothing we do is independent of these. We cannot do anything in our lives without other people being involved, despite how much you think you are an independent free soul! Just getting some bananas requires a societal monetary system that trusts and honours your transaction, someone to grow and gather bananas, someone to distribute bananas, and someone willing to sell you bananas.

For this reason, I emphasize that we always need to consider the *resources* humans strive for, the things we actively try and get and do, and at the same time always consider the *social relationships* through which we get all these resources. The two always go together because we do not get or do anything in this world without other people. When you analyze a particular social relationship, you need to find out what is done with that relationship—not in a mercenary way but just what naturally flows or might flow from that social relationship.

In this way we can consider our very 'selves' and our life histories to be made up of many resource-social relationship links or pathways. When you buy a banana, you need a social relationship with someone who sells bananas (unless you grow your own, and then you need different types of social relationships). This social relationship will be what sociologists call a 'contractual' relationship, or what others call a stranger relationship, which usually works because of monetary reciprocity (in a western capitalist economy that is).

So, what are 'internal states' and 'inner worlds'?

What has been called our human 'inner world' is a mixture of two things (Chapter 1). First, part of this is merely a trick for explaining human behaviour when you do not really know what is going on (you have not explored contexts). This has always occurred ("He did that because he was angry") and is even done with inanimate objects ("My car didn't start because it was angry with me getting up so early"). This is even called "the fundamental attribution bias" by social psychologists, but they attribute the 'cause' of using this bias to something inside of people, such as faulty cognitive processing, which cannot be seen, thus showing the same bias themselves ironically (Edwards & Potter, 1993).

But the most refined versions have occurred since the late 1800s and were developed initially by medical people who were given the task of explaining unusual behaviours they could not understand (Guerin, 2020a). For example, the 'causes' of those behaviours they labelled as 'hysteria' were shown to not be physiological, so they eventually 'explained' them by saying they were 'psychological', an abstract and invented term, which appeared in the late 1800s (Guerin, 2020c). In many ways, the whole of psychology has been built and developed by assuming the 'cause' of people doing things we do not understand must reside 'inside' them (Chapter 1). From a social contextual perspective, these medical people did not know how to look for the social and societal contexts which were shaping these 'hysterical' behaviours all along.

The second part of what is meant by the 'inner worlds' of humans is far more real and important and is about *the behaviours of talking and discourses*. A great part of what humans do is to respond to all events in their lives with words, even if not directly related. This is because our social relationships are essential for everything we do in life. Whatever events are going on, and however we might respond to those events, we also respond with a lot of words and talking. Such words and talking, however, are not superfluous or epiphenomenal, because they have very real effects on the people around us—they are an integral part of our lives and how we manage our lives (more in Chapter 7).

The only difficult part to understand from all this is that the responding to our worlds with words and language does not originate 'inside' us and is not contained 'within' us. It is difficult to see where our words are coming from, so we again make the fundamental attribution bias and assume there is an 'inside' person constructing sentences, applying grammatical rules somehow, etc. But such behaviours are like any behaviours we do and are shaped by the worlds we live in as our bodies engage with that world—in this case our *'discursive' worlds*, all the talk and writing around us, which has been going on since we were born. But because we cannot easily see the social and societal bits of our worlds, which have shaped all these words (because we could be responding to a person who is 10,000 kms away), they have been 'explained' as *originating* somehow, somewhere, 'inside' us. But our ways of talking and the forms of talking are learned from all the myriad of discourses around us as we grow up, and then further shaped and nuanced by more local resource-social relationship links in our lives.

So, the two parts of the 'inner' worlds of humans go together, and we can use the new analysis to pull apart their use in therapy discourses. One is about explaining events we cannot observe or understand by saying they must be originating inside us somewhere. The second is all about responding to social events, or the social consequences of non-social events, by using words and language, and we will see in the next chapter that 'emotional' responses also fall into this category. These two facets go together because when we cannot easily see the social worlds which shape our talking, we 'explain' them as something originating 'inside' us.

I will say more later in this chapter and in the next about the special cases of *thinking, consciousness* and *emotion* and how they fit into all this. I hope you can begin to see why all these topics and the (supposed) explanations have been confused for centuries. This is because they are real behaviours involving words (talking, thinking, emotions) while engaged in worldly events with real consequences. The trick, however, is that they are not actually shaped by those worldly events themselves but shaped by our social and societal worldly events which might not even be present at the time. This gap between our thinking or consciousness and what we are doing at the time (one does not cause the other) has led to a lot of confused discussions.

I will try to illustrate these now because they are difficult points to get a strong feel for. Imagine you are painting your house. You are being shaped by the walls and paint and the effects of seeing the colour go onto the wall, etc. But at the same time, you are usually doing a lot of talking, but probably not out loud (= thinking, Chapter 7). This talk might be *totally unrelated* to what you are doing (something that happened with your kids earlier in the day, or something you have to explain to your boss on Monday). But it can equally be related to the painting, but—and here is the gap I mentioned—*this thinking or consciousness is not shaping your painting*; such talking or thinking we might be doing concurrently is about *social responses* most directly relevant to your social relationships (my parents will hate this shade of blue I am using; if the paint streaks I will look a fool).

So, the problem here is assuming that your talking, thinking or consciousness is shaping what you are doing—in this case painting. It does not shape your painting, *but neither is it epiphenomenal*, it is extremely important *social* responding that we always need so we can deal with our social relationships.

So, our 'consciousness' is our talking and thinking about events going on in our life and these can and will directly affect our social relationships, *but they do not control what we are doing*. My 'consciousness' of my painting is real talking or thinking and is not epiphenomenal, and it might affect what I say later that day or how I excuse my shoddy painting, but it is not directly controlling the painting I am doing. The *social contexts* of such talk and thinking might eventually influence my painting, but not directly.

Possibilities versus 'facts' or 'knowledge'

One thing to learn about contextual analyses is that they mostly look for *possibilities* rather than certainties. The idea that words can be true or false is an old one which needs changing (Guerin, 2021). What contextual analysis tries to do is to generate many and varied possibilities for examination (Guerin, 2016b). These can then be tried out by doing things in the world or making observations; they are never confirmed by saying more and more.

What this is getting at is that the only things certain (or true?) in this world are things we do, not things we say. We can observe things wrongly, but assuming we double check with more than one observer, *the things we do might be called 'true' but not the things we say about them*. So, there can only be certainty in what people do and this includes *that* people are saying things. If someone says, "There is a cat" then *that they said this and the social effects can be certain* (if we observe well), but what they said cannot be true or false.

This is a difficult starting point, which comes out of discourse analysis and some postmodern thinking. Truth is in doing; verbal knowledge can never be certain or true; we can only be certain that somebody did say something and observe the effects it has. We will come back to this and how it affects the way we view 'mental health' later in this chapter, but the problem is that a large number of the 'mental health' behaviours are talking or thinking. To get you prepared for this ahead, talking is not about saying true or false things; talking is about doing things to other people—it is just one way of doing all our social behaviours. Talking (and thinking as we will find), do not have special extra properties, no special properties of truth or anything else, they are just behaviours that we do, which can affect other people as part of our normal social behaviour, and the effects they do have will shape us in turn. They are, however, a very specialized way of doing all our social behaviours and that makes them special in another way.

So, the aim of contextual analyses is to observe people's contexts because that is what shapes what they do. From this we generate *possibilities* of what might be going on, and we can then 'test' those by *doing* something to the world and seeing what happens, not by giving more and more words of 'support' to try and prove it is true. Guerin (2016b) gives some guidelines to help you generate possibilities.

Finally, you should treat this whole book in this way. What I am doing as an author is to throw up lots of possibilities for analysis and rethinking of 'mental health' and therapies *to get you to do and say things in new ways*. I am not presenting you with facts or truths, but with ways to explore what is happening in these bad life situations.

Language behaviours

Obviously, both language and non-language behaviours are important for any analysis of human life, but language behaviours are of special importance for the analysis the 'mental health' and therapy behaviours. That is why I will spend all of Chapter 7 dedicated to this topic. This will include both thinking and emotion, as you will find out (both are behaviours that are part of language use, as it turns out), and many of the 'mental disorders' are about poorly shaped language practices resulting from a history of poor social relationships.

The importance of a thorough analysis of social relationships

The final point to discuss before getting into the analysis of 'mental health' behaviours, is about the importance of doing a thorough analysis of social relationships. I have already suggested that humans only get resources through social relationships (R-SR), but this also means that we can only sustain social relationships by exchanges of resources (in a very broad sense). Our relationships give us some things directly, but they also give us opportunities for other events and things in the future, give us opportunities to tell stories stemming for our relationships for others who are in other relationships with us, for fun, enjoyment, etc.

This analysis means that we must consider a wider range of 'social relationships' than psychology typically does. In modern society, we have many more social relationships with strangers and people we rarely see, and these different forms of reciprocity and ways of continuing the relationship and making exchanges, with these different forms of reciprocity and obligation have very different social properties to those of friends and family (Guerin, 2016b). Sociologists have long explored such 'contractual' or 'stranger' relationships, and they make up a large per cent of our total social relationships in modern life, so they are important to analyze. They are also likely to lead to 'mental health' behaviours about anxieties, since with contractual relationships both parties have no responsibility or obligation beyond the contract itself, meaning that such relationships are built on a tenuous link.

These forms of relationships and their connection to modern 'mental health' issues will be explored further in this book (Guerin, 2017, 2020c). The other point to make here, however, is that the predominance of contractual relationships also means that the different parts of our lives have become very fragmented or 'compartmentalized'. This simply means that it is easy to keep the different resource-social relationships completely separate in modern life, so our family do not know what we are doing at work or with our friends. Again, this has social properties of what we are able and not able to do.

We can learn a lot about all these changes in modern social relationships from sociology, as I have done, and these are important to know when working in therapies. We learn less in this case from social anthropology, simply because social anthropologists have traditionally worked in more isolated groups and communities in which everyone is known to each other, and they are mostly related as kin in some way.

Is SCA just doing the same old thing, changing some old abstract words for some new abstract words?

The final point for this chapter is that looking at human behaviour in its contexts has the strong advantage that all these contexts are potentially observable. If you suggest that a person did X *because* of their low self-esteem, you cannot observe that (Chapter 1). If you place 'self-esteem' in its full contexts, it becomes a way of talking (and acting) which has been shaped in particular social, societal, discursive, and cultural contexts; and these contexts and this shaping are observable, at least potentially. Even thinking and consciousness, if considered as talking shaped in discursive communities, but which has been punished for being said out loud (Chapter 7), can be potentially observed. We can also potentially observe how societal structures can shape (usually by limiting opportunities) both talking and therefore thinking.

The catch here, of course, lies in the 'potentially'. The traditional methods of observation and research in psychology do not give us any potential for observing such concrete shaping, and this is why the discourses of psychology have been abstract and attributed to events 'inside' the person. But using new methodologies allows such observations to expand, methodologies which not coincidently were developed within the other (contextual) social sciences

(Guerin, Leugi, & Thain, 2018). These are the observation and research skills not taught to psychiatrists and psychologists, which has led them to not see what is shaping human behaviours, and which have then led them to attributing 'cause' to an abstract and 'hidden' world.

References

Edwards, D., & Potter, J. (1993). Language and causation: A discursive action model of description and attribution. *Psychological Review*, 100, 23–41.

Guerin, B. (2001). Individuals as social relationships: 18 ways that acting alone can be thought of as social behavior. *Review of General Psychology*, 5, 406–428.

Guerin, B. (2016a). *How to rethink psychology: New metaphors for understanding people and their behavior.* London: Routledge.

Guerin, B. (2016b). *How to rethink human behavior: A practical guide to social contextual analysis.* London: Routledge.

Guerin, B. (2017). *How to rethink mental illness: The human contexts behind the labels.* London: Routledge.

Guerin, B. (2020a). *Turning psychology into social contextual analysis.* London: Routledge.

Guerin, B. (2020b). *Turning psychology into a social science.* London: Routledge.

Guerin, B. (2020c). *Turning mental health into social action.* London: Routledge.

Guerin, B. (2021). From "What is philosophy" to "The behavior of philosophers". *Behavior & Philosophy*, 48, 69–81.

Guerin, B., Leugi, G. B., & Thain, A. (2018). Attempting to overcome problems shared by both qualitative and quantitative methodologies: Two hybrid procedures to encourage diverse research. *The Australian Community Psychologist*, 29, 74–90.

7 The pivotal role of language for life and therapy

If you wish to understand 'mental health' and therapy, you need to have a major rethink about language—what it is, and what it is for. Language is intertwined in all the conundrums and puzzles of these topics and if you cannot sort language out properly, you will continue to go around and around in metaphorical circles—replacing one way of talking with another but treating it as a breakthrough (Figure 1.1). This cycle has been going on long enough.

As a starting point, all the 'inner' worlds, mental states, mind, psyche, cognitive processes, consciousness, experience, etc. are all just about talk. There is no inner world of humans—there is no person inside looking out. These are all ways of talking that involve metaphors, imagery, and sometimes persuasive storytelling. They are very real and useful ways to talk in everyday life (see below), but they are *not* reports on something or some state 'inside' us. (As we will see below, they mostly refer to discourses which have been punished when said out loud).

If you understand that last paragraph you will glimpse why understanding language is so important (Guerin, 2020a, Chapters 3 and 4). To emphasize this, here are some more links we will make:

- language is just a way of doing our social behaviours and social relationships
- the most important thing about language is *not* the words
- the most important thing about language is how it affects other people and our social relationships
- language is not about saying things but about doing things to other people
- language can have no effect on the world other than on people
- language produces some unique social properties
- the unique social properties of language can be both very good and very bad

So, what we will discover is that it is when social relationships break down that a person's language use also breaks down, and this means that all the 'language disorders' and 'thinking disorders' are really 'social relationship disorders' (including societal relationships). And to fix these 'disorders' we need to fix a

DOI: 10.4324/9781003300571-9

person's social relationships and the uses of language within those. We will also find that when a person's language breaks down this also means their uses of language to plan, concentrate, remember, answer questions, etc. become problematic as well. Over the next chapters I will develop ways to find out a person's 'discursive history' and their discursive relationships and communities.

To stretch your rethinking even more:

- thinking is also language use, just the bits which are not said out loud and which therefore develop their own special social properties
- emotions are also either a form of talking ('emotional discourse'), or
- emotions are substitute behaviours when we *cannot* speak (for many reasons) but must still respond

So, I am going to spend a lot of time on how you can understand people by the contexts they are living in rather than by finding more and more new words with which to talk about a fictitious 'inside' person. This is because so much of therapy, therapeutic talk and theories, and the process of therapy is about talking and discourses, and we need to get to the real bottom of such talk, and not assume it originates from 'within' as our 'causal' explanations suggest. In this way, a lot of therapy talk and theories just go around and around in circles with more and newer sets of words.

This might be fairly confronting for some therapists, since the common frame is that the problems are 'inside' the person and need to be talked through to make things change. But you need a good understanding of language and its uses, like we saw for the 'proxy' foundations of behaviour in the last chapters (self, emotion, inner person, etc.). If you assume mainstream versions of language, you will not understand its roles in current therapies and therapies for the future.

Some basics of a contextual approach to language use

The main feature of language use has already been given—that it is just a behaviour we do that can affect other people and thereby affect us as well, and that we can do almost all our social behaviours using language (not quite all). Our focus on any language use therefore needs to be on these analyses: *what is this talking or writing doing to other people? What is it accomplishing for the speaker's social behaviour and life? (and it could be avoidance or escape, remember).*

Answering these questions is the whole area of discourse analysis (Guerin, 2016), which tries to fit what someone says into the to-and-fro of their social life, not to autonomous 'processes' in their head, and this is what we will need to do with all the talking and thought 'disorders' claimed by the DSM (Chapters 3 and 9). If you are sitting with people and someone says, "I heard a funny story the other day", you do not analyse this in terms of their cognitive or brain processes, but in terms of what is this doing in that group conversation for that person who said it and what it has done previously. It could be they were trying to maintain the friendships with a humorous story, it could be they were embarrassed by the silence, it could be they were trying to distract the conversion away from a topic that was punishing for them, or it could be that the funny story itself was about something more direct for one of the people present.

In life we use a lot of language to manage our resources and social relationships, and these include telling stories, giving explanations, giving excuses, making jokes, bonding, planning, and following instructions. These behaviours all appear in therapy in exaggerated forms, but we must remember that our focus should be on: what is this piece of language use doing to the listeners, and what consequences does it have?

Let me comment briefly on some common forms in which language gets used in life, and which get broken when our social relationships do not work. Remember that these are really analyzing changes to social relationships (using language) not analyzing the words or grammar or such things. Also remember that in therapy situations these can apply to the discourses the recipient has in their 'home' environment, to their reporting of their life events to the therapist, to the therapist's talking to the recipient, and to the interaction conversations occurring during therapy.

First, there is everything that is currently called 'cognition' within psychology, and all of *the events we call 'thinking'*. I will deal with these in detail later in this chapter as they commonly seem different (and they indeed have special properties compared to language spoken out loud). For example, everything we call 'memory' or recall is really about language use, and therefore inherently depends on the social context, not on whether it is true or not. These forms include thinking, consciousness, discernment, hearing voices, and rumination. "I feel like everything I do is wrong".

Second, there are *uses of language to get people to do things directly*. Common forms in our lives are friends and family asking (or demanding) that people do things, and perhaps just as commonly people at work (colleagues and other stranger relationships) getting you to do things for your job. As we will see later, all these change over time depending upon the social relationships and histories involved. Many of course are not bad forms of 'demanding' but good forms: "Can you help me do this and I will help you in the afternoon?" They all need the right contexts of some reciprocation to succeed (Guerin, 2016).

Third, there are more specific forms of the previous point, which are common when *using language to get people to do things through written rules*, and which are enforced (words need the social relationship consequences to have any effect, remember) through corporations and businesses where you work, law courts, governments, police, civil service, schools, colleges, and universities, etc. These are the bureaucratic forms [sic] enforced through government or corporate social consequences (Guerin, 2020b, Chapter 1). "You cannot do that because the rules do not allow it".

Fourth, there are *forms of talk which purport to be directly reporting about the world* and its consequences with the (purported) aim of letting listeners follow these (true) rules about the world to do things correctly or save them from bad consequences. What they get you to do might be to say certain words or act in some way. These include science statements, medical stories, lectures on anything, and all the myriad ways we *explain* things to other people in everyday life and present our *beliefs* (Guerin, 2020b, Chapter 5). "It would be easier if you did it this way".

Fifth, there are the forms which are there mainly (or completely) *to manage our social relationships*. These can be weird because the content of what is said is not the important thing about such uses of language, just that it is able to enhance or manage a social relationship. But at the same time, they are not frivolous or useless because if we do not manage our social relationships (whether kin, friends or strangers), then all our resources will fade away and our other talk will have no effects anyway. So, whereas such talk as rituals, jokes, and gossiping might seem frivolous; they are important. Such forms also include all the entertaining talk and the community-entertaining talks. On the larger scale we have literature, novels, poetry, oratory, songs, and theatre. We also have ritualized talk, myth telling, other forms of storytelling and narrative, Indigenous and spiritual knowledges, rumours and gossip.

I will include a sixth category (since I do not really believe these categories are distinct anyway) of *talking about who you are and your life plans and goals.* There is a lot of such self-talk done in life, but this is not really a direct report of your 'self' but a mixture of doing things to people to have them do things (our first and second categories above) and also of managing your social relationship because you are telling these stories about yourself. So, it is a mixture but is frequently used to deal with your social relationships (Guerin, 2020b, Chapter 5). "I'm the sort of person who likes going for walks in the bush". This statement could have all sorts of effects depending on the contexts in which it is said.

All these forms get mixed up, but whether they work or not, as I keep reminding you, depends on your social relationships and the context—not the words themselves. The situation of a government trying to enforce the words, "Do not drive over 50 kph here", is very different from saying to a friend, "Can you pass me the salt?" But both are real and can have consequences.

Why is this important to specific 'mental health' behaviours?

I will insert a little more about 'mental health' and therapy here, to hint at its relevance. I have already written earlier that many or most of the 'mental health disorders' arise from language not working in the normal way, and that this arises from issues with our social relationships, personal as well as societal social relationships. When language messes up then a lot of our behaviours do not work anymore (do not have any effects), and collateral problems occur (more in Chapter 9). As a heads up, here are some examples of those problems, put into a very general form:

If you exaggerate storytelling, you appear delusional

If you exaggerate the use of language for planning and rationality, you appear with anxiety or obsessions

If you exaggerate the joking and dramatic functions of language, you appear 'crazy' or manic

If you exaggerate the uses of language to keep distance from people, you appear to have 'word salad'

If you exaggerate the many avoidance and exiting strategies which use language, you appear with depression or 'negative symptoms'

While I will not go through all the discourse analysis details here, there are four important topics which need to be covered so you can make sense of the analyses of 'mental health' behaviours throughout the rest of this book. These are:

- language disguised as non-language
- general or specific references in discourse
- thinking
- emotion and its weird relationships with language

Language disguised as non-language

When we do things and engage with our worlds, most of what we do is certain (true is not the usual word we use for this). I eat an apple and I make the bed. We can be messed up in our observations but with reasonable observations, especially by more than one person and repeated over time, doing things is usually fairly certain. Some observations are trickier, if there are quick movements or things are hidden, but apart from this, doing things is reasonably certain.

But when we use language and words, on the other hand, this is also certain but only in the sense mentioned earlier: that what I say and what effects this has on other people, we can observe fairly well, at least within the same limits of observational clarity as any other doing things. Using language is just another form of doing things but with the proviso that it only ever can do things to other people who have learned that same language. So, if I *say* "I ate an apple" this is a very different event with different contexts, different consequences (social only), and different observations needed than just eating an apple as an action with no talk.

The problem is this: people have always wanted to claim that 'what language says', or the 'meaning' of the words, can be more or less certain, ranging from a property called 'truth' to another called 'falsity'; assuming that hearing words are sort of similar to observing actions. After centuries of thinking this way, I am now here to debunk this (following many earlier philosophers and others). You need to start thinking of language (and later thinking and emotion) as just behaviours we learn socially and which *can* do things to the world, but only to other people, not to cats and chairs and cars. And *saying* "I ate an apple" can have important social effects irrespective of whether you ate an apple or not.

This clears up a lot of philosophical-type questions which have been around for centuries and never solved (Guerin, 2021). They have never been solved not because no one has got the answer correct, but because the question was wrong in the first place. "How can a sentence be true?" is a bad question. A sentence is just a behaviour we learn to say or write because of the effects it has had *on other people*—it is never true, nor is it ever false. It just is. It is something we do which can change what other people do.

Now, the reason I am spelling this out is that for a few centuries at least, people have tried to claim the same certainty in language that we have when I drop a vase and it smashes on the floor. Not certainty that I said or wrote something, but certainty in a fictitious property called 'meaning' or 'truth'. We can observe someone pick up a cat and that is fine, depending upon how well our observations were made. We can also observe someone say, "That is a cat", and observe how people respond to that, and this is fine depending again upon how well our observations were made. We heard them, or even recorded them, saying this and perhaps also observed what other people around did— what effects did it have? But it is a totally different and fictitious idea that we can then assign a property to this sentence, "That is a cat", and claim it is also 'true'. It is just something we did out loud. We are constructing something out of nothing. Just as eating an apple has real effects, so saying a total falsity and getting strong reactions from people is having a real effect.

The problem with this is that *people try to disguise language use as non-language doing so that they can claim the certainty for their uses of language*: "My poetry is better than yours!" "You have a personality disorder". They can make sentences *seem* true and powerful even though they are not, and it is only ever the social relationships (what listeners do when they hear you) that gives our words any effects. Trying to call some sentences true is really a bluff.

To help you work through these disguises, Box 7.1 has some ways to decide whether you are dealing with uses of language or not. This can also be useful in therapy when deciding (analyzing) whether what is said by the other with certainty is just words or not:

Box 7.1 Tests to give you a clue that words are being used as shaped strategies (behaviour which is shaped by audiences) rather than simple descriptions of the (non-word) reality (behaviour shaped by the consequences of what the world does to you).

Ways to tell simple descriptions from complex persuasive uses of language.

- if it is abstract it is probably a word event
- if it is generalized it is probably a word event
- if it is active it is probably a non-word event

- if it is concrete it is probably a non-word event but there are social strategies in which concrete verbal descriptions are used as a ploy to make it seem more real (Potter & Edwards, 1990)
- if it is singular or specific it is probably a non-word event
- if you repeat the behaviour over and over, are the effects like repeatedly hitting a wall with a brick or does the repetition produce other effects, more like the effects you get from people when they are bored or exasperated?
- if it can be easily said, or can be said clearly, then it is probably a word event
- if it makes a good story, then it is probably a word event
- if it needs a lot of arguments rather than observations, then it is probably a word event
- if you need to be convinced of it then it is probably a word event
- if the person is looking towards other people during the behaviour, then it is probably a word event; if they are looking towards the relevant environment during the behaviour then it might be a non-word event
- imagine the person reporting this in front of a judge and jury; would it hold up?

An example. If someone says to you, "No one I know likes me", it is fairly clear that this is a complex language use and not a simple description of 'fact' (although it is disguised to make it look like that). For discourse analysts, the sentence is *abstract* and *generalized* across many people, so it clearly cannot be a simple description. This means that it must be analyzed very differently. If it were a simple description ("Mary threw a rock at me"), then we would need to look at this person's world and what happened with Mary. On the other hand, as a complexly shaped language use cunningly disguised as a simple description ("No one I know likes me"), we need to find out how the person has been shaped to say this, when clearly they cannot justify the abstract generality of it—*what audiences in their bad life situations have shaped the person to say this? What does saying this do in their bad life situations? Does saying this help in some contexts of their life?"* So, the sentence itself is therefore directly about this person's social relationships! And remember that this applies to therapists' talk as well (Chapter 3).

General versus specific

A very important point to learn for clinical analysis is whether the behaviours have been shaped by *general* or *specific* contexts. This might not seem important at first (many of my students do not get it at first) but becomes extremely important. Given that almost all human behaviour of clinical interest is socially shaped, we have possibilities that the behaviours were shaped only by specific people in the person's bad life situations, or it could be the cumulative shaping from multiple social groups and society as a whole (including people never met). The difference between "My friends do not like me" versus "No one likes me" is big; they are shaped by very different contexts and need different ways to handle them.

Generalized or abstract social relationships are ones commonly:

- shaped by everyone the person knows (unlikely unless you are living in a very bad life situation)
- shaped by less people but the person is living in a socially restrictive world, so these people *are* their total social world
- shaped by *societal* restrictions and punishments (patriarchal, colonial, lack of societal opportunities, bureaucratic, governing, mass media, social media)

Following the previous section on distinguishing language from non-language use, generalized shaping will often be noticed by the use of 'extremes' as defined by discourse analyses: everyone, everybody, never, always, no one, nobody, them all, shameful, etc.

To give an example, a person engaged in research with me spoke about the first time they opened up to someone about their childhood abuse, after being silent about this for more than 30 years. They saw a television news headline about a high-profile arrest for child abuse and reported that the first thing they thought when seeing this was, "Oh no! Now everyone will know (about me)". So, it was not that their parents or spouse might now find out about them, nor their specific friends, nor even the perpetrator; their shaped response was that now *everyone* will know about them. The real point is that this needs to be analyzed and treated differently.

I will come back to this distinction throughout this book since it determines a lot of how we might support people in distress. For helping and healing people, this means a good deal of contextual questioning over people's social relationships, being prepared for the possibility that there might not be one or a few people who have made life a problem for this person, but whole systems and society itself, but the person has not been able to escape this shaping or find an alternative way of living outside of the mainstream.

There is a worse problem here, however, that should be mentioned now. We can have issues and conflicts with life and solve them. More often, however, our life issues and conflicts can become 'language events' rather than conflict events. So, someone might take some money of mine and this is an issue and needs to be resolved. But those events are also likely to become 'language events' by being *told* to a number of other people, including the person who took my money. *Our material life problems usually also become discursive problems.*

The real issue here is that one of the properties I mentioned earlier for language, is that language is not shaped and maintained by the events themselves but by how our audiences respond—the discursive consequences not the material event consequences. This means that *once a material issue becomes a discursive issue it will be more difficult to change or stop it occurring*, since it is not just a matter of getting the money back, but of influencing and changing all those audiences who have been involved in the 'discursive event'.

This is the basis for most of the 'anxiety' issues. Whatever the named material events talked about in anxiety, the real events now have become discursive ones which cannot be changed just by resolving the material issues. The audiences are still there for the new discursive events. So, the worry, planning, obsessing and rumination continue unabated, no matter what happens in the material sense to the problem. This means that anxiety, rumination, and obsessional problems, as well as problems with beliefs and delusions, require discursive changes to be made, not changes to the objects and events which are being named in these discourses.

The reason I bring this up here is that if the discourse gets a general or societal audience then this becomes worse. "No one likes me" cannot be talked out by showing the person that one person likes them, since this is not a general discursive issue. Likewise, "I am the King of England" cannot be talked out by showing (materially) that the person is not a king, since this is a discursive problem. In all cases, changes to the person's discursive communities and contexts will need to be made with the person (cf. Guerin, 2003).

Later chapters will address this problem and what we might do to help. In Chapter 9, for example, we will see that even when a person's bad life situation is cleared up, there have been consequences of living in that bad life situation which continue, and the person does not seem to be able to just 'get over it'. A lot of these 'legacy' effects are due to a problem becoming a 'language event' and especially when these have been shaped into being general or abstract uses of language.

Thinking, and the supposed 'inner world' control of behaviour

Analyzing thinking follows from what has been said above, but with a few important differences. Thinking consists of the same discourses, stories, phrases, and words we have learned in our lives for doing things to people with our words, all of which are about managing our social relationships. Anything we do in life or confront in life, we have learned to respond to using words as well as any other responses. The difference with thinking is that it is all the *talking responses which are not said out loud*. In essence, thinking is just our talking we have learned to do in any situation to manage people, but not done out loud. It is still an engagement with our material social worlds (since language only has effects with people) and does not originate 'inside us'.

So far, so good. But this analysis of thinking shows some differences to talking, and these are important for practical work with people in therapy, especially since a large percentage of the 'mental health' behaviours are about language or involve language, and many have been labelled as 'thought disorders'. Since thinking is really about managing our social relationships via language use, therefore *'thought disorders' are also really 'social relationship disorders'*. (Except that these are not 'disorders' but ways of managing life through very bad life situations. We will come back to this in Chapter 8.)

Table 7.1 gives some possibilities as to why someone does not talk out loud. Why are they thinking something rather than saying it out loud? These are really useful in practical settings for assisting people who have problems with their 'thinking'. Some are innocuous, such as not having another person present at the time, whereas others are more important, such as the person having most of their talking in life punished by other people (Freud's *repression* is an example).

So, your first analysis when working with someone presenting their thoughts to you, whether this is yourself or another person, is to question why this was thought and not said out loud. Is that minor or does it reveal something very important? This was Freud's major breakthrough, that by using various

Table 7.1 For all the verbal responses we have been shaped to say in any situation, not saying them out loud (thinking) can arise through the following ways

- if there are simply too many learned verbal responses for the context you are in to 'say' them all ("What do you think of modern art?") Simply put, you can only say one thing at a time, even if you have a lot of possible responses in that context.
- if there is not enough time (if there is a busy conversation and you cannot "get a word in edgewise"). This is one reason thoughts *appear* to occur more when you are alone, *even though they occur whether or not you get to blurt them out loud.* You can just observe them better if alone.
- if a verbal response has been learned in a very specific context (my friends are talking about fast cars but the one relevant story I know only makes sense to my family), so I do not say it out loud because it will be punished. But I 'think' of it still (it has been shaped) and could report this afterwards if asked whether I was thinking of that story during the conversation.
- if there are no audiences present for the verbal responses (if I am alone perhaps). In such situations it can be suggested that the verbal responses *which normally occur across a large range of my audiences* will be the ones reported if you are suddenly asked "What are you thinking about?" I can also, of course, talk out loud without an audience present if this has not been punished, as sometimes occurs.
- if the verbal response has been punished in the immediate social context before (but might be said out loud in another social context). "I bit my tongue", in common English slang.
- if the verbal response has been punished in most contexts ('repressed'?) so that I might need special forms of questioning to remember afterwards that I was even thinking it (it was afforded in that context); people who are typically silenced
- if saying out loud will be punished (so they remain only as thoughts) because different audiences in your life have shaped *contradictory* verbal responses which you can only safely say out loud in one group or the other but not at the same time
- if the verbal responses or discourses have been shaped by very generalized contexts so that when I would respond there is no clear or concrete audience for this (shaping by 'sociological' discursive communities: media, patriarchal, economic, colonizing, bureaucratic). *"I am so angry at this whole social system but who do I yell at?"*

'therapeutic methods', he got people to say out loud some thinking (talking) that they had never before said out loud. He found that in many of these cases those thoughts would have been severely punished by those around if they had been said out loud. The problem was that Freud did not know how to explain this, so he invented some 'inside us' pseudo-explanations, which proposed that something 'inside us', 'the unconscious', originated these thoughts. We can dispense with all this jargon and yet still theorize and keep the main observations which Freud made; that people had verbal responses about the social relationships in their lives which would be punished if they said them out loud, so they did not say them. But these verbal responses were still present as 'thinking'.

So, the first thing we can glean from listening to people's thoughts is the analysis of why that talking was not said out loud. When looking at how we might change a person's discursive communities, there will be clues in what they are thinking and the audiences who punish such talk.

Thinking also appears a little different to talking out loud in another way. This arises because there are no immediate social consequences for thinking, since there are no social relationship changes happening at that time which are shaping your world on the spot, and this is different than when we are talking to someone face to face. This means that *some features of face to face talking disappear when we are thinking our responses.* Table 7.2 shows some of these.

The primary difference is in grammar. Grammatical consistencies function to make our language use fast and accurate when talking to someone. If we did not use grammar our language could still function, but it would be slower and less accurate. The more we think (talk but not out loud), the more our thoughts (and eventually speech even) will lose grammatical features and the other features in Table 7.2. People trying to live in bad discursive communities will lose their grammar, even when they do get to talk out loud. It will come out as 'telegraphic' speech.

So, the points in Table 7.2 are therefore important for another reason, beyond just explaining how thinking works. In some cases of 'language

Table 7.2 With no listeners or consequences, the thinking afforded in any context is likely to change in these ways from speaking out loud.

- lose a lot of grammatical features
- be shorter
- you would probably also not continue your thinking as a real conservation because there is nothing/no one to react—there is no 'turn-taking' to shape what you say next (but you will get to think more of the responses you have)
- your thinking therefore will appear more as phrases or 'snippets' of conversational discourses rather than as whole sentences, compared to talking out loud
- any physical persuasion effects (staring wildly at them in shocked disbelief) might disappear as well (but sometimes we grimace and smile on our own)
- the thinking also becomes unmonitorable and this can have both good and bad properties, and might change what is said/thought; you might 'think' worse things than you would ever have said out loud, even though both were occasioned by the same scenario; you might say ruder things about the person in the third scenario than the first two scenarios, in other words …

disorders' these same features arise. When you hear these, they are a clue that *the person's speech is not being shaped by strong social relationships anymore*. You can look for these same features not just in thinking, but also in spoken patterns for someone living in bad life situations. Check the person's total range of relationships in their life. These will also arise in Chapter 9 when we look at why, when a trauma is finished and over with, that a person cannot just 'get over it' but there are still bad contextual effects happening to them.

Emotion and its weird relationships with language

Emotion has always puzzled psychologists, and people in general. Our emotions seem to spring up at odd times when things are chaotic or distressful. The term 'emotion' includes a lot of behaviours which barely seem connected, such as crying, laughing, anger, despair, screaming, loving, fright, anxiety, etc. Are these really all related?

There are a large number of theories and a whole lot of (futile) attempts to find out how many emotions there really are. Most theories see them as a reaction, usually somehow ill-defined as being 'instinctive' or 'hard-wired', to stressful or contradictory situations. That sort of makes sense then that when trying to survive in bad life situations, people would show a lot of emotion. But are they really 'instinctive' behaviours? Many of these appear in what therapists say about therapies (Chapter 3).

One clue is the century-long and inconclusive dispute between two types of theories. One says that when we are in, say, a frightening situation such as being chased by a dangerous bull, this causes emotional behaviours such as being scared and being scared causes us to do something useful, like run and get out of there. So, this is said to prove that we evolved to have emotions because they are useful for survival (although maybe not in the modern world which has only a certain type of bull). The other side of this pointless dispute says that the scary bull causes us to run (this is the instinctive bit they say), and the running causes us to then be afraid. So, in this case the emotion is a later behaviour, although it is not clear why we would have this emotion.

Taking a contextual look at emotion we can see some of these bits are probably right but maybe not for the right reasons. First, a lot of what is *labelled* as 'emotion' is simply the use of language to do things to people; "I am getting angry, please stop doing that". These have been called "emotive discourses" (Guerin, 2020a). But there still is another variety of what is called 'emotion' when chased by a bull, that of being scared. But clearly, we are not 'being scared' to persuade the bull to stop chasing us.

My way of reconciling these very different behaviours – all called 'emotions' – is two-fold and represented in Figure 7.1:

- some are a language-based phenomenon plain and simple ("You have really upset me now"); we use discourses about 'emotion' to get people to do things or manage our social relationships like any words (whether successful or not)

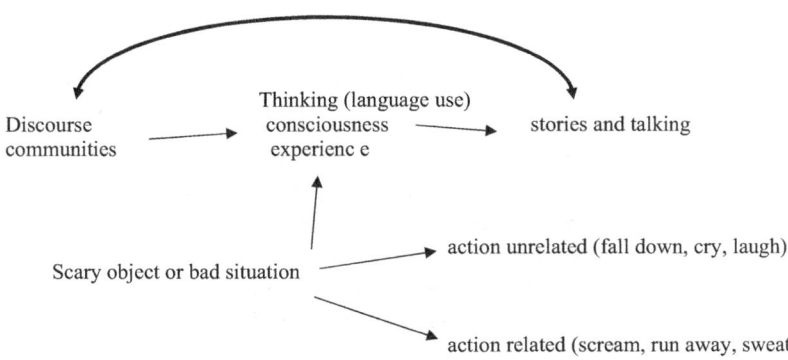

Figure 7.1 Contextualized 'emotions' in scary situations. At the top is 'emotive talk', when we just talk about the situations we are in as our response, but this is really about our social relationships and not dealing with the dilemma situation.

- the second type of 'emotion' (crying when upset or being scared when chased by a bull) is *related* to language use but in a different way. When we deal with difficult situations, we normally do this by using language, except when being chased by a bull (although you might curse the bull as you run away); emotions in this sense are what we do *when we cannot use language to respond* but we still need to make some response (usually for other people)

So, the second type of emotion, then, consists of behaviours we do when we have no other (functional, context-specific, learned) behaviours, *but we need to say or do something*. These emotions have these conditions:

- situations in which we have no already-shaped responses (we usually respond in life by 'using our words' so emotions will be typical when we cannot use words to change things, or when there are *no possible words that would work*) and
- these situations require us to respond in some way (usually to escape bad consequences, but also when overwhelmed by enormously good outcomes or in new or too complex situations)

In particular, we will see that a common situation is some intense event for which a response is required *but you have no words*, no responding with language (since saying something is our everyday response we can do almost anywhere, anytime). Box 7.2 shows some of the life situations which can lead to emotional behaviours and being asked to answer difficult questions when in a crisis will fall into this.

Box 7.2 Life situations which might show a lot of emotional responding.

- have very bad outcomes (bad life situations)
- have unexpected outcomes (normal response not appropriate and you have no language available for that reason also)
- have multiple but contradictory powerful outcomes
- be new situations but which are highly consequential
- are social situations since these are often difficult to disambiguate for people
- be situations in which there has been no prior learning of what can be done
- be consequential situations in which there are no language responses possible
- involves a person with little life experience of learning multiple and flexible responses
- the person cannot *see* anything shaping their behaviours such as societal shaping of behaviour (see earlier section on *General versus specific*)
- the person has limited language use or their language use has been proscribed

Which behaviours a person actually does in such contexts depends on the person and their contexts, obviously. Many of the 'emotional' behaviours are common behaviours and *appear* 'instinctive' but this is only because they are behaviours which are (1) *always available* and (2) *which do not need words*. This is also why the same behaviours, such as crying, can be found in both happy and sad situations when there are no obvious language responses, but a response is required all the same.

Why is this important? For trying to help someone showing 'emotional' behaviours, we must explore the contexts for these behaviours, as always. For example, if someone bursts into tears, do not think that they are having an instinctive response to a bad situation, but explore these questions:

- have they learned crying as a way of doing things to people? (emotional discourse)
- what is the distressful situation they are facing for which they have no other responses?
- why can they *not* talk about the distressful situation as their response? What is happening there?
- what is the contradictory, new or baffling situation for this person?
- what responses do they *not* have that *other* people might do in the same situation? What would *you* do?

- what might they do in this situation other than the emotional behaviours?
- what are the hidden contexts they cannot see?
- what social relationships might be involved since for these it is usually difficult to see what might be a correct response because they are so convoluted?
- why do they need to make a response at all? Why can they not just be silent or quiet?
- is my very questioning of them as a helper (forcing them to give a verbal response) the problem here? Am I forcing them to make some form of response when they actually have none to give?
- if they have an emotional response do not then make them talk about their emotions or 'feelings'; they probably responded in that way *because* they have no words

These figure widely in therapy situations when people are dealing with difficult problems that cannot be easily talked about (or they would have solved them before). Once we learn more about what are the life situations which shape the range of 'mental health' behaviours (Chapter 8) you will see better how these 'emotional responses' are important and how they can tell you things about the person's context that need following up.

References

Guerin, B. (2003). Combating prejudice and racism: New interventions from a functional analysis of racist language. *Journal of Community and Applied Social Psychology*, 13, 29–45.

Guerin, B. (2016). *How to rethink human behavior: A practical guide to social contextual analysis*. London: Routledge.

Guerin, B. (2020a). *Turning psychology into social contextual analysis*. London: Routledge.

Guerin, B. (2020b). *Turning psychology into a social science*. London: Routledge.

Guerin, B. (2021). From "What is philosophy" to "The behavior of philosophers". *Behavior & Philosophy*, 48, 69–81.

Potter, J., & Edwards, D. (1990). Nigel Lawson's tent: Discourse analysis, attribution theory and the social psychology of fact. *European Journal of Social Psychology*, 20, 405–424.

Part 3

Rethinking 'mental health' as living in restrictive bad life situations

8 Contextual models of 'mental health' behaviours

Behaviours shaped by restrictive bad life situations

Many people like and repeat the quote by Victor Frankl (2006): "An abnormal reaction to an abnormal situation is normal behavior". This implies that people with 'mental health' symptoms are reacting in an 'abnormal' way, but they are reacting to an abnormal situation. This takes the blame off the person for their behaviours, so they are not pathologized. The same idea was many years later echoed in this quote, while researching some of the contexts which shape the 'borderline personality' behaviours:

> We conclude that practitioners need to explore a greater range of contexts for any symptoms, and that rather than thinking of individuals in terms of *having* a 'borderline personality', we suggest rethinking of them in terms of *having had* 'borderline socializing environments'.
>
> Fromene & Guerin (2014)

If we think of people's behaviours, talking, thinking, and emotions as being shaped by their *external contexts*, rather than originating inside of them somewhere (Chapter 6), how do we contextualize 'mental health', therapy, and healing? To do this properly we would need to know a lot about the social, societal, economic, patriarchal, colonized, historical, and cultural contexts in which people are embedded from birth. But psychiatry and clinical psychology do not do this when assessing people. Everything is explained as originating internally, inside the person somehow and somewhere; whether this is 'personality', 'brain physiology', 'chemical imbalance', or 'faulty cognitive processing'. We saw in Chapter 1 that these all fall for the 'fundamental attribution bias'.

More pointedly, if we are to get rid of the DSM as a diagnostic 'tool', which has come to narrowly define 'mental illness' research and practice, and to begin depathologizing psychology and psychiatry, then the Frankl quote above is a good place to start (as are Allsop, Read, Corcoran, & Kinderman, 2019; Bentall, 2006; Caplan, 1995; Davies, 2014; Guerin, 2017, 2020a; Johnstone, 2014; Johnstone & Boyle, 2018; Kinderman, 2019; Watson, 2019). This also follows a contextual approach for redefining the very foundations of psychology and psychiatry (Chapters 6 and 7; Guerin, 2020a, 2020b, 2020c).

DOI: 10.4324/9781003300571-11

So, when the question is posed: 'But what are we to use instead of the DSM?' the answer lies in the Frankl quote and the different contextual approaches. Instead of defining people by a non-scientific category system (Davies, 2014), which pathologizes what they are doing, saying, thinking, and feeling, the answer is to *spend more time observing people as individuals and their contextual worlds* and to answer the following questions idiosyncratically for each individual in distress (rather than put them in new categories):

- what are these 'abnormal' situations that Frankl writes about?
- what are these 'abnormal' reactions that Frankl writes about?

To which a contextual approach adds:

- how do these 'abnormal' situations function to shape these 'abnormal' reactions? (and what other behaviours do they shape?)

This is the substance of the present chapter, from which we will move next to contextualizing therapy. In this chapter, I want to start answering these three questions in a general way, then we will look more at specifics and how that determines the help we might give to people. Forget the DSM categories and focus on the behaviours and contexts that have shaped them.

What bad life situations shape the different 'mental health' behaviours?

What are the life contexts or situations for people who have developed 'mental health' behaviours at some point in their lives? Luckily, we know a lot about this from the writings of those with first-hand experience, and from the observations of many professionals who care for them (and do more than just categorize). When you stop attributing problems to something pathological 'inside' a person, you also begin to observe more carefully the situations in which they are living. A plethora of bad life situations become apparent, but these extend beyond the 'abnormal reactions' we currently call 'mental health'.

Box 8.1 has the main bad life situations (Frankl's 'abnormal situations') listed, which shape the 'mental health' behaviours we can observe (Frankl's 'abnormal reactions'). A useful task is to go through each of these and try and get a feel for what your life would be like living under those conditions. What would you, or could you, be shaped to do, in order to cope, survive, or just 'put up with' things as they are? If the situation continued or got worse, what 'abnormal' behaviours (Frankl) would you start doing to cope? Frankl (2006) thought this through based on his life experiences living in a German concentration camp during WWII, but the same behaviours get shaped with many other bad life situations (cf. Todorov, 1997; Turnbull, 1973). A similar list can be found as "threats" in the power threat meaning framework (Johnstone & Boyle, 2018; also see Bloomfield et al., 2021).

Box 8.1 Common forms of 'bad life situations' which can shape the 'mental health' behaviours

violence and living in a violent or bullying environment

forced displacement in war or environmental catastrophes

crime and living in criminal environments

unemployment, bad jobs

long-term drugs habits

death of close family or friends

poverty

lack of opportunities, or silencing

traumatic events of all sorts, long term or short

strong restrictions imposed on behaviour so there is little real choice, even when no overtly 'bad' events occur

many behaviours become blocked completely by severe imposed restriction

oppression and violent control taken by individuals or groups

abuse of all sorts: physical, sexual, power, control

exclusion or discrimination from social relationships

combat and fighting of all sorts, especially if trapped in or restricted to violent situations

having disabilities or less flexible behaviour repertoires which restrict opportunities

the person does just not 'fit in' the world they were born into

bullying over time, especially at school, work, in family

many bad situations occur through hospitalization itself and through medication

Something that will become apparent throughout, as we discover the origins of 'mental health' behaviours in these bad life situations/contexts (and not inside the person), is that these situations occur for many people. You might recognize some from your own life, but not all of them will shape long-term or chronic 'mental health' behaviours, however. Following the Frankl quote, most people will find *other ways* of dealing with, surviving, putting up with, or escaping such bad life situations. I will come back to this point and later, point out some specific life contexts which will shape the 'mental health' behaviours, which occur when a person *cannot* escape in some other way.

Most of these bad situations are easily observable situations when anyone bothers to observe them, but there is a plethora of other bad situations which are not at all obvious unless very careful contextual observations are made, and unless the observer has developed their 'sociological imagination' (Mills, 1959). By this is meant a whole range of social, societal, patriarchal, colonizing, and cultural practices which all shape our behaviours, but which are not immediately observable. So, while forms of violence and abuse can potentially be observed, if they are not kept secret (but which they often are), the effects of, say, a competitive capitalist economic system, living in tight nuclear families without external monitoring, or a constant need for marketing your 'self', are less easy to observe even when you try.

As sociologist Sam Richards (n.d.) said:

> My students often ask me, 'What is sociology?' and I tell them, 'It's the study of the way in which human beings are shaped by things that they don't see'.

Someone, then, with a good 'sociological imagination' (Mills, 1959) can meet a person, listen to them talk about their life situation, and become aware of many potential or 'possible' (Guerin, 2016) societal shapers of their behaviours, which the person themself might not even know (and they therefore often blame themselves or a physical person in their world). Psychiatrists and clinical psychologists are *not* trained to have sociological imaginations and so 'mental health' behaviours are instead said to originate inside the person somewhere, the mistaken attribution error.

> By some historical accident, the study of the unhappy or disturbed personality has been assigned to physicians, perhaps the least equipped of all investigators of man to deal with the problems. Unlike others in the biological sciences, physicians have next to no training in scientific methodology, and—more important—*they are trained to look for causation in the organism rather than the organisation.*
>
> (Arnold Rose, 1962, p. 537, my emphasis)

Below are a few of these 'less easy to observe' bad life situations which arise from the way that our modern lives are now run (Guerin, 2016, Chapter 3 of 2020a). They are difficult to observe without training and appropriate research methods (Guerin, Leugi & Thain, 2018), but they are very real nonetheless and have very real effects:

- we are being restricted into economically useful but socially not-always-useful nuclear families with little outside monitoring of what happens within the family, even when the people are loving
- our families are busy and driven by the economic system we live in, and have little spare time to listen or be supportive
- if our nuclear family is not supportive then there are few others who can be, unless they are paid (stranger or contractual social relationships, including therapists)
- our lives are filled with strangers who have no obligations or responsibility for us outside of the contracts we have (the paid carers go home when the money stops)

- we are governed by societal rules we did not make or agree to, but we are still punished when we err
- our society is built (economically and socially) on the idea that we are all self-contained individuals who can choose our own life options and can be blamed when we do not succeed
- because we are assumed to be self-contained individuals, our society is built on the idea that every individual is therefore responsible for what happens to them and can be blamed for anything going wrong (implicitly or explicitly blamed)
- we are being forced into life activities which are 'marketable' for employment (and hence resources) but which we would never choose otherwise
- we are forced to survive in bureaucratic systems that are too complex for most people to navigate
- other life options we might do get blocked off because of societal limits on opportunities (the gross inequalities of modern societies)
- other life options we might do are blocked off because all life options require money or some other capital
- when traumatic events occur, the responses are not monitored by others
- when traumatic events occur, we no longer have close social connections who can help us; we need to arrange paid care
- we live in a competitive world because our economic system is based on this, which increases the bullying and lack of real social connection

Those trying to help or care for people with 'mental health' behaviours need to be aware of, and sensitive to, these sorts of *modern* bad life situations. These need to be included in any therapist education.

Which behaviours get shaped in these bad life situations?

We have now seen a range of bad life situations which correspond to the 'abnormal situations' in Frankl's quote which started this chapter. However, when we ask the question of what behaviours get shaped by these bad life situations, the answer turns out to go well beyond the 'mental health' behaviours. It is clear from both research and experience that such bad life situations listed above shape a massive variety of behaviours. Figure 8.1 shows some of these in five very broad categories.

So, there are many possible life strategies to cope with, survive, put up with, or avoid bad life situations, and this should not come as a surprise except that 'mental health' has been staked off into a world of its own and *'owned'* by the medical models, in a territorial way, for over 100 years. In most bad life situations, people probably do something small to change their situation and life works out okay. I might lose my job, which potentially is a bad life situation given our reliance upon money for doing everything and anything in life now. But I might get support from friends and people helping me find new employment and I can cope with this. I do not go into crime and I do not

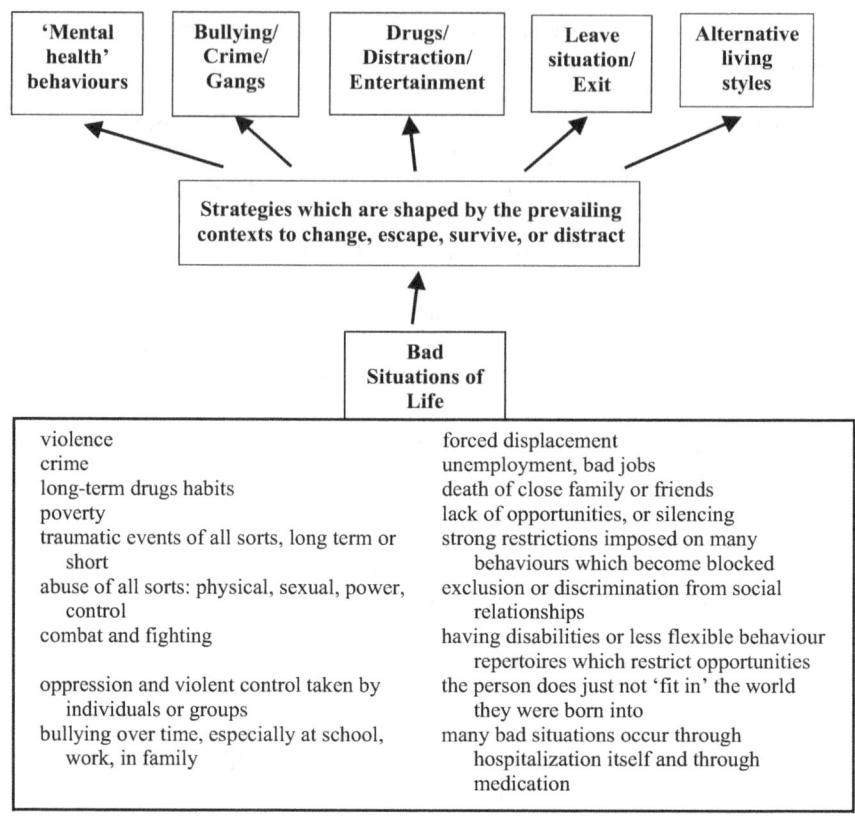

Figure 8.1 The behaviours and strategies which can be shaped as ways of coping with, surviving, putting up with, or avoiding bad life situations

develop 'mental health' behaviours (I probably do get shaped into some but not to a 'dysfunctional' level).

But some people move into delinquency or crime to try and change their bad life situations in which they find themselves; they might gain new social relationships and resources in this way to get out of the bad situation. Others 'put up with it' but use distractions and entertainment to avoid the worst impacts of their bad situations and wait for contexts to change over time. Others find ways to just leave, perhaps by going and living elsewhere or moving in with friends (cf. Hacking, 1998). And still others might settle for an entirely alternative ways of living, to leave their bad life situation ("Get thee to a nunnery!"), even to the extent of becoming homeless for periods. And most life strategies include a mixture of these (Agnew, 2005; DeNora, 2015; Feinberg, 1996; Hartman, 2019; Hewett, 2004; Matza, 1969; Mayo, 1969; Nordhoff, 1966/1875; Tolokonnikova, 2018; Wacquant, 2008; Watkins & Shulman, 2008; Wyatt-Brown, 1988).

This raises some interesting and important points.

1   Which of these strategies actually happen for any particular person will depend upon a number of contextual features of their life, not something internal to them. We will return to this in the next section since the main concerns for this book are *those specific conditions which shape the 'mental health' behaviours rather than any other 'abnormal' responses.*

2   We would expect any person to have been shaped over time into more than one of these 'solutions' or strategies for their bad life situations. Indeed, for a few years now, whenever I have been talking to people with first-hand experience of the 'mental health' behaviours, I have also asked them about the other possible strategic solutions. In almost all cases they report having tried some of the other ways, but that they did not work out (the contexts were not right). So, it is not that drug taking 'causes' mental health behaviours, or that heavy metal music 'causes' mental health issues for metalheads; but rather, that people are trying a variety of possible solutions to survive within their bad life contexts (Rowe & Guerin, 2018). [As a caveat to this, I will mention below that those who are shaped into 'mental health' behaviours will *also* have been shaped into a number of *other* 'mental health' behaviours as well. No one ever has a single and permanent 'mental health disorder'; they have been shaped into multiple solutions to their bad life situations. Having a series of 'mental health' behaviours shaped is probably the norm, in fact, but is disguised by the DSM.]

3   I have only listed very broad categories, and more nuanced research and practice should be able to discern how the behaviours observed for any individual were functional in trying to deal with their bad life situations (but not necessarily beneficial in the longer term). There will be many variations on all of these, and multiple strategies will probably have been tried, so there is no point trying to lump everyone into only one of my five broad categories.

4   This means that there will be closer connections than currently recognized between people working with human difficulties such as 'mental health', homelessness, crime and delinquency, drugs, alternative groups and living arrangements, etc. What connects these groups, professionals or not, is not some similar disease of the brain, but the same bad life situations which have shaped different strategies to find something better for life. This means that we should be able to begin pooling the expertise of these groups (including first-hand experiencers, carers, community workers, forensics, psychologists, psychiatrists, mental health nurses, social workers) and find *new ways to solve the bad situations, regardless of the presenting* behaviours (whether delinquency, 'mental health', drugs, etc.). This might coincide with such areas also looking for new ways forward (Maylea, 2021). I will come back to this point in Chapter 11 when looking at how therapy might be done differently in the future.

How contexts and behaviours are intertwined

Which of these different life solutions or pathways get shaped, will depend on the person's contexts, their life skills, and their social relationships and resources. Figure 8.2 presents some general ideas of how this might occur for shaping the behaviours and pathways for 'mental health', bullying and crime, distraction, escaping or exiting, and taking up alternative lifestyles. 'Mental health' will be discussed in the following section, however.

None of my broad suggestions are meant to be sweepingly true statements. Rather, like 'mental health', the situations and strategies shaped by them *need to be contextualized for each individual* as everyone will have slightly different life contexts. Contextualizing means observing, listening to them tell their story, and using your own background experience to come up with *possibilities* that are then discussed openly with the person and observed where possible

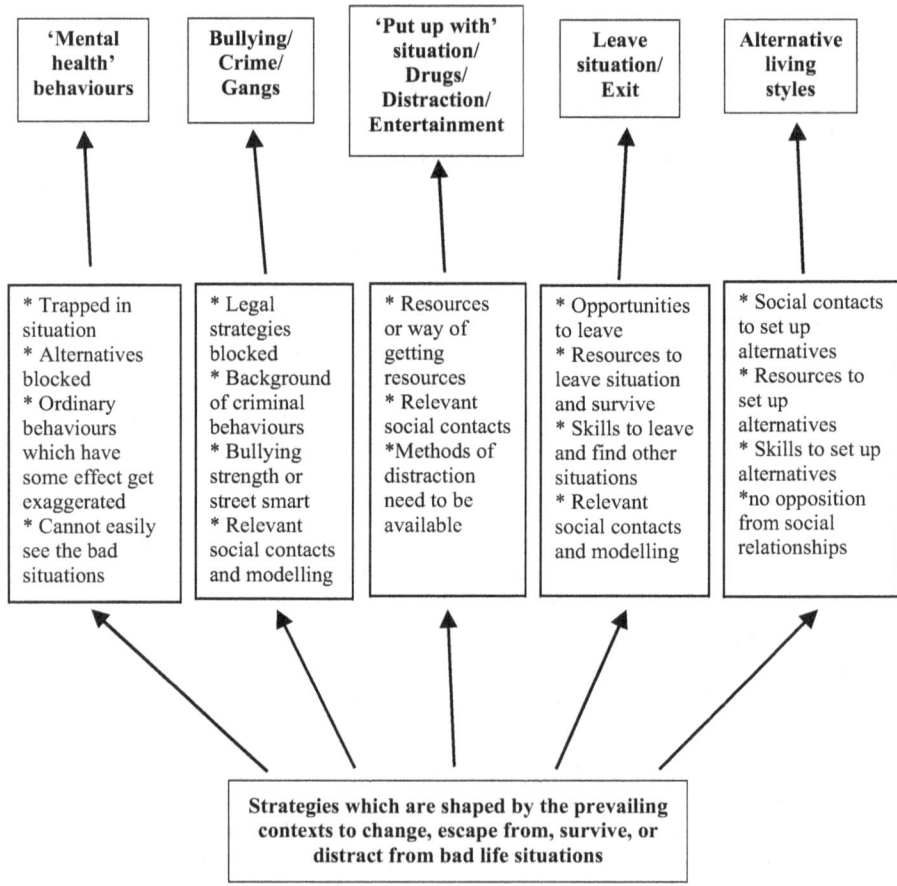

Figure 8.2 Behaviours and strategies shaped by living in bad life situations

(Guerin, 2016; Mills, 1959). We do not need yet another categorization system brought into existence.

Crime and bullying. For example, if a person is in a bad life situation of some sort, they can find ways to escape this by non-legal means (Adler & Adler, 2012; Belknap, 2007; Cullen & Agnew, 2003; Dahrendorf, 1979; Damousi, 1997; Decker & Van Winkle, 1996; Mayo, 1969; Truong, 2018; Wardlow, 2006; Yablonsky, 1962). If other alternative but legal means are blocked by people or by governments, then this route is more likely. However, to do this, there need to be contexts in place. If there is a family or social network history of delinquency or crime, then the person will have had modelling on how to make this work—you need social contacts and skills to make this work (it is not genetic!). There are also probably a whole group of 'petty criminals' *who were shaped into crime but were not very good at it* and ended up doing lots of small and risky strategies. I have heard of some who find prison a good escape from bad life situations (regimented and free food), and do not mind prison because it provides escape.

Distraction and entertainment. There are multiple ways of distracting oneself from our bad life situations, including entertainment of many descriptions, drugs, risky behaviours, excessive behaviours, and forms of comedy (cf. Hartman, 2019; Wyatt-Brown, 1988). There are also music, dance, literature, and arts (Rowe & Guerin, 2018). These are all really ways of 'putting up with' bad life situations, or 'making the most of it', as is said in English. People still need resources and social relationships to make most of these events happen, however, and some of these 'solutions' have long-term consequences which are not beneficial for the person (such as certain drugs).

Exiting. Escape and exiting bad life situations are always possible responses, but these also require some skills, resources and social relationships to make them happen. Suicide can be thought of as one 'exiting' solution for some people. (In this way it is very different in most cases to self-harming.) But it still requires some resourcing to carry out and usually is intermeshed with social relationship conflicts. People are also known to just leave when things get too bad, and even to return later (Hacking, 1998). Military service is another way, with many vets reporting that they joined the military to get away from their home situations.

Alternative lifestyles. Finally, we can consider that some people 'discover' or 'are converted' in moments of bad life situations to alternative lifestyles than the one causing distress. This ranges from religious conversion during bad situations (James, 1958/1902; Nordhoff, 1966/1875), to joining alternative lifestyle groups, to moving to a more peaceful rural or coastal lifestyle (sometimes called a 'sea change' in Australia), or just moving away to a new beginning with a loved one or friends. People with refugee status are another group, although they might have been *forced* into exiting with no real plan or control over where they would end up. Many others explore alternative ways of behaving and living life *without engaging with the mainstream of society which is the source of their bad life contexts* (Brill, 2008; Cohen, 1971; Cohen & Taylor, 1976; Eckert,

1989; Glasper, 2006; Goodlad & Bibby, 2007; Hewitt, 1997; Nordhoff, 1966/ 1875; Orwell, 1933; Rowe, 2018; Sartwell, 2014).

All these strategies have many finer nuances, but crime, bullying, drugs, distractions, exiting strategies, and a strategy of pursuing alternative lifestyles, all:

- require both resources and social relationships (even for refugees)
- require some life skills, which many people will not have
- have no guarantee they will succeed any better or for very long
- can have longer-term deleterious effects, which might even be worse than the original bad life situation (e. g., drug escape leading to addictions and poverty)

These changes can be useful for those who have been shaped to the 'mental health' behaviours, and recommendations for clients to find a totally new life situation (as their therapy) have previously been used in psychotherapy (e. g., Haley, 1973, 1985). But it must be remembered that advice is one thing, and finding the resources, skills, and social relationships to make these alternatives work is another. Too many people end up merely *talking* about leaving and exiting strategies, while in reality they 'put up with it' for the rest of their lives.

The important point from all this for 'mental health' is that the behaviours of 'mental health' are just that, behaviours. They are specific ways of behaving that have been shaped by specific bad life situations, but which could have turned out otherwise depending upon a lot of life conditions. 'Mental health' behaviours, in this way, are nothing special or unique except by their conditions of shaping (see below). We need to stop thinking about them as being exotic, or in another time and space, hidden 'deep' and 'inside' people, and see them more as Frankl did. Whether they occur or not depends upon the specific contexts of living in a bad life situation, not on a brain, chemical or cognitive dysfunction. The latter are false internal attributions arrived at because the context has not been examined closely.

The specific shaping of the 'mental health' behaviours by bad life situations

What, then, of the more specific contexts which shape what are currently called 'mental health' behaviours? Figure 8.3 shows the major contexts in which bad life situations will shape some of the 'mental health' behaviours. As mentioned, usually more than one have occurred over time.

The four main contexts for bad life situations to shape 'mental health' behaviours are these:

- the person is trapped in their bad situations, which are often very restrictive or oppressive. This means that other alternatives are not possible, and they must 'put up with' the bad situations.
- any possible alternatives behaviours and life strategies are blocked, usually by social or societal relationships. Other alternatives are usually actively blocked and usually by other people or societal 'rules'. Even in a

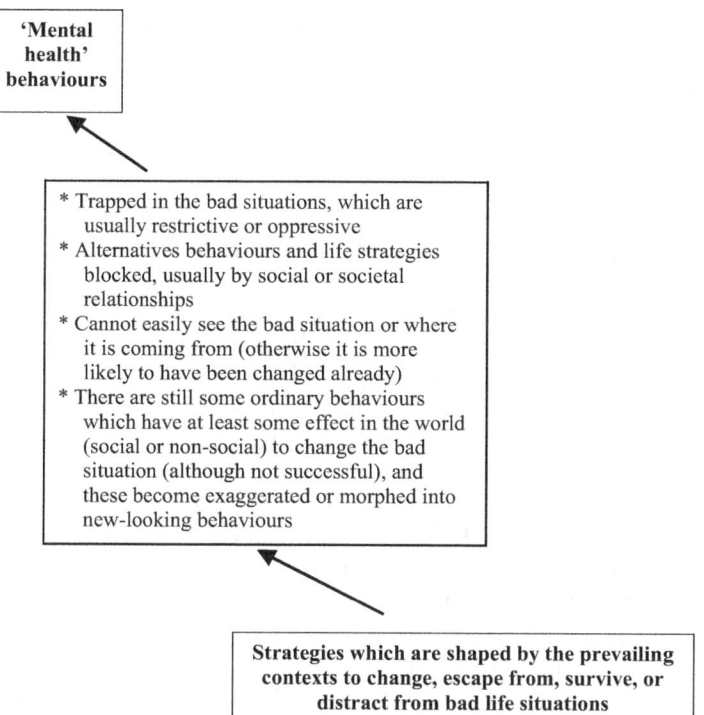

Figure 8.3 'Mental health' behaviours and strategies shaped by living in bad life situations

superficially loving family who say they care, alternative ways of behaving can be actively blocked for the children's 'own good' or 'because we care about you'.

• the person in the situation cannot easily see the bad situation or where it is coming from (otherwise it is more likely to have been changed already). This can be from societal restrictions on behaviour (e. g., patriarchy shaping what both men and women are allowed to do), or from disguises and secrecy, such as a superficially loving family who nonetheless block alternative behaviours.

• the person can still do some ordinary behaviours which have at least *some effects in the world* (social or non-social) to change their bad situation (although not successful usually), but these ordinary behaviours will become exaggerated or morphed into new-looking behaviours, which now appear 'abnormal'. These other behaviours are usually ones which require few resources or social relationships to engage (such as self-harm) but can still lead to some effects in the person's world (however futile).

The behaviours shaped by bad life situations having these properties are the ones currently called 'mental health' behaviours.

In these ways, the contexts are different to the earlier given strategies to deal with bad life situations, since the person in this case cannot do them, as they are restricted and trapped in some other way. Obviously, people doing other strategies can also have more intensive periods where what they are trying to do is thwarted (crime, escape, etc.) and so they might well be shaped into some of the common 'mental health' behaviours for periods along the way which might fluctuate. Again, this all means that people can go in and out of 'mental health behaviours', depending upon the current contexts, and in and out of the other strategies as well (crime, escape, etc.). *The singular attribution of someone having 'a mental health disorder' or not is wrong, as is the whole of idea of making a 'diagnosis'.*

These extra contexts can occur across the whole population not just those less privileged. Those living in wealthy family environments can just as easily be restricted and trapped as those in poverty, although how this plays out will differ as you listen to individual stories. For example, being wealthy means that resources are available for people to do more escape or alternative lifestyle solutions, of course, and more resources for buying drugs, but it also means that rich families will restrict the behaviours of members so as not to risk losing their capital. Being in poverty contexts is very restrictive in different ways, especially in modern society for which money is a prerequisite for doing *any* life strategies (and even for getting help from a professional).

As another example, abuse itself does not necessarily lead to these 'mental health' conditions. But there are concomitant effects of abuse which change all the other contexts of life, and lead to major life restrictions and the other conditions which shape 'mental health' behaviours. Indeed, we know that childhood abuse predicts *both* later behaviours currently labelled as 'psychotic' and also later criminal activities (Johnstone & Boyle, 2018; Malvaso, Delfabbro, & Day, 2016). Different solutions depending upon the contextual outcomes.

This means that we do not need another category system of 'mental health' but rather *we need methods for observing and listening to people in distress to find out their idiosyncratic bad life situations and the range of attempted solutions they have been through.* This is the first part of helping people who show 'mental health' behaviours: listen to their stories and get the details in a broad way of the bad life contexts in which they are struggling; find out what they have done already; find out what did not work out and the missing contexts; what has been restricting them? what happened when they tried something new?

What are the 'mental health' behaviours?

Our next point of departure is to examine the behaviours which get labelled as 'mental health' behaviours, as a result of being shaped in the more specific contexts previously listed (Figure 8.3). This is surprisingly difficult for a number of reasons. Most importantly, almost all the behaviours are not completely 'abnormal' as Frankl wrote, but turn out to be everyday, ordinary behaviours, but which are usually (1) exaggerated, (2) done in situations which are not usual, or (3) morphed into slightly new behaviours. In that sense Frankl still is correct, they are mostly 'abnormal reactions', but the basic behaviours making up these reactions are not brand-new ones appearing from nowhere.

So, we all need to start thinking about and observing such 'mental health' behaviours—whether doing, talking, thinking or feeling—as normal behaviours that we all do but which might have gone wrong somehow because of abnormal life situations. The behaviours themselves are easy to find, so long as we do not try (again) to categorize them into fictional 'diagnoses'. As mentioned in Chapter 1, I take seriously the observations and engagement of therapists and others, but do not take their explanations or category systems seriously. To this end, I have used the observations from the DSM while eschewing their category system and their explanations in terms of diseases and faulty cognitions.

Box 8.2 gives a list in alphabetical order (to stop you trying to recategorize) of the main behaviours listed in the main DSM-5 categories (APA, 2013). These were cut and pasted directly from the DSM (Guerin, 2017). Some are still a bit abstract, but they will do.

Box 8.2 Alphabetical list of the main behaviours to be found in the DSM diagnoses.

acute discomfort in close relationships

generalized anxiety

opposition behaviour

affective instability

grandiose ideas

orderliness preoccupation

agoraphobia

grandiosity

overactivity

anxiety, appear anxious or fearful

grossly disorganized or abnormal motor behaviour

overestimating threat

appear dramatic, emotional, or erratic

hallucinations

over-importance of thoughts

appear odd or eccentric

hopelessness

panic attacks

argumentativeness

hypersensitivity to negative evaluation

perception disrupted from normal

attention seeking

identity disrupted from normal

perfectionism

being awake throughout the night, decreased sleep

impulsivity

perfectionism preoccupation

being reckless

increased alcohol and drug use

phobias

body representation disrupted from normal

increased energy

preoccupation

cognitive or perceptual distortions

increased physical health complaints

problems in the self-control of emotions that brings the individual into significant conflict
concentration difficulties
increased sex drive
racing thoughts
consciousness disrupted from normal
increased spending
rapid speech
crying spells
inflated sense of responsibility
recurrent and persistent thoughts
defiance
intermittent explosive anger
repetitive behaviours applied rigidly
delusions
intermittent explosive behaviours
repetitive mental acts applied rigidly
desperation
intermittent explosive irritation
restricted range of emotional expression
detachment from social relationships
interpersonal relationships instability
sad mood, sadness
disorganized thinking
intolerance of uncertainty
self-control problems that bring the individual into significant conflict
disregard for the rights of others
intrusive and unwanted thoughts
self-image instability
distrust and suspiciousness of others' motives
irritability

sleeping troubles
disturbance of eating, or eating-related behaviour
lack of empathy
slowing down of thoughts and actions
dysfunctional beliefs
lack of enjoyment, loss of interest in pleasurable activities
social inhibition
eccentricities of behaviour
memory disrupted from normal
somatic changes that affect the individual's capacity to function
emotion disrupted from normal
moodiness that is out of character
spending less time with friends and family
empty mood
motor control disrupted from normal
staying home from work or school
excessive emotionality
need for admiration
submissive and clinging behaviour
excessive fear and anxiety
need to control thoughts
suicide thoughts
feeling overwhelmed
negative symptoms
unable to adjust a particular stressor
feelings of inadequacy
nervousness
worry
finding it hard to take minor personal criticisms

Have a glance through these, now they are separated from the purported groupings of the DSM. See how many of them *you yourself* have done at times, but: probably not for long; probably only in situations in which they were deemed 'appropriate'; possibly in a joking way; and probably only in a mild form.

Now imagine what life situations could happen to you, *really restrictive bad life situations*, that might make you do these for longer, or more intently, because they still get some effect out of people when nothing else you do can. This is the way we can start to think about such 'mental health' behaviours when we observe them in chronic and exaggerated by people. Stop assuming that something inside the person has gone wrong—brain, chemicals or 'cognitive processes'—and look to the bad life situations which might have shaped such intense and exaggerated actions out of common 'normal' behaviours. We need to spend more time finding out these contexts and placing the causes 'internally' is just a quick way to avoid having to carry out that step. Instead, listen to the person's story, ask for details, and observe them as much as you can *in situ* rather than in an office.

Which behaviours get shaped under the specific 'mental health' conditions? (How might we regroup these behaviours into more functional groupings?)

What is required for the behaviours to be shaped and maintained?

While the behaviours shaped for humans living in bad life situations will be idiosyncratic and depend on the possibilities within those idiosyncratic situations, some guidelines for thinking of possibilities are useful for those working with people in distress. A friend once described this to me as like blowing up a balloon, especially those long thin balloons. As more and more stress is put on the balloon by blowing into it, some natural and induced weaknesses will appear so that at some point along the balloon a new swelling or 'blister' will bulge out—a normal section of the balloon gets exaggerated! What determines that exact point depends upon a lot of detailed contexts. Here are four guidelines for which common mental health behaviours might appear when under the four extra contexts of bad life situations:

Behaviours which appear to the experiencer to have an effect to change the situation. For the person in very bad life situations, there are behaviours which *appear* to have *some* effect to change the situation, irrespective of whether they actually succeed in either the short or long term. For example, any form of withdrawal or escape, or behaviours which could lead to withdrawal or escape, will occur and get exaggerated even if not immediately successful; all the 'depressive symptoms' and 'negative symptoms' are examples of these. Also, any behaviours which *appear to be solving the situation* will likewise be shaped in normal and exaggerated forms; constant thinking, anxiety, and perfectionist behaviours are examples. As a more extreme example, delusions are stories which can appear to have effects by engaging listeners, and the types of stories shaped (real delusions) are actually perfect for engaging mostly disinterested listeners but usually exaggerated too much. There are many other examples we will come across during this book.

Behaviours which can be done with almost no resources or social support. Many of the common 'mental health' behaviours are simply behaviours which (1) can appear to have an effect in the world to the experiencer *and* which (2) do not require any resources or anyone else to support the behaviours. Examples are crying, self-harm, withdrawal (depression, negative symptoms), disrupting food routines, excessive rumination (anxiety), and spontaneous violence. For example, key *contextual* features of self-harm are: that it does not require anything much for it to occur (in this way it is unlike suicide); self-harm requires minimal equipment; self-harm can be hidden and kept secret up to a point; and no other people need to be involved in carrying it out (as opposed to some other risk-taking behaviours). As another example, we always have food preparation, serving and eating, even in most bad life situations, so *interrupting these* in any way can also be done without resources or people and can have *some* effect to change your world (albeit not successfully in the long run); so, behaviours of refusing food, being fussy about food, excessively talking about your food, excessively eating food in a way not shaped by hunger, etc. will be shaped into exaggeration.

Behaviours dependent upon local contexts and past histories. While the behaviours in the category above were singled out because they do *not* require resources or social support, most of the 'mental health' behaviours listed earlier do require some. Sometimes these just need modelling or social responses by others. To use an example of reacting to stressful situations with violence or bullying, some persons with limited behaviour repertoires (often labelled with 'mental disabilities'), will frequently react in distressful situations with a reactive flailing, which can be violent to those around, but those around will be sympathetic and try ways to reduce the effects in the least restrictive ways (since restricting makes another bad life situation). However, other people in bad life situations who have had the effects of violence on those around *modelled* before, will likely have more nuanced violent or bullying behaviours shaped when under duress (taken from the alphabetical list of Box 8.2, these could variously include: argumentativeness, being reckless, defiance, disregard for the rights of others, eccentricities of behaviour, grossly disorganized or abnormal motor behaviour, violent hallucinations, impulsivity, increased energy, intermittent explosive anger, intermittent explosive behaviours, intermittent explosive irritation, irritability, moodiness that is out of character, opposition behaviour, perception disrupted from normal, problems in the self-control of emotions that brings the individual into significant conflict, racing thoughts, rapid speech, recurrent and persistent thoughts).

Behaviours which could be random or new after 'sampling' several other different strategies. Finally, some of the behaviours could appear random, meaning that the exact detailed contexts are probably not traceable, even though real. It was also suggested earlier that most people in distress will not react with a single behaviour, but will have a variety of responses shaped, most of which might disappear after having seemingly no effect on their world. So, in some cases, these mixtures can generate new varieties or combinations, or at least more nuanced versions of the original 'ordinary behaviours' which were shaped into exaggeration.

Important conclusions

There are three important points for listing these guides to understand how 'mental health' behaviours are shaped from living in bad life situations.

- The first is to help you to break away from the DSM groupings and narrow ways of thinking and analyzing into categories.
- The second is to warn you *not to over-interpret the behaviours themselves*. So rather than thinking that self-harm is really a way of getting revenge on the self you dislike, think instead about self-harm as an 'abnormal reaction to an abnormal situation', which is done because it requires few resources or social support—it is easily done and easily hidden, and *appears* to have an effect to change the person's bad life situation. The real point here is that these behaviours arise in different ways from trying to live in unliveable situations, and we can understand how these behaviours might have been shaped, but the real point is still to try and change that person's bad life situations.
- Third, in terms of prevention, there is a lot more that can be done about recognizing bad life situations and trying to change them *before* they get to this stage. There is also a lot more that can be done to recognize early forms of these behaviours, perhaps transitory ones, which again indicate that a bad life situation remains and needs to be changed.

What functional groupings might we try?

I have found that once we dispense with the DSM groupings, we can begin to see new connections between the many behaviours. We must remember, as pointed out above, that those experiencing distress from bad life situations might show several of these, changing over time. I believe that this is missed when people are too focused on getting a DSM 'diagnosis'. And there are ways that such interconnections, which do not follow the standard DSM, become hidden or disguised:

- they are currently *hidden* within the DSM by following the large range of 'comorbidities', which cannot be ignored under the pretence that they are independent diagnoses just because the DSM says so
- they are currently *hidden* within the DSM by the huge overlap in actual symptoms between 'independent' disorders that are diagnoses (now

revealingly called 'transdiagnostic' symptoms), which is 'corrected' by a large listing of 'differential diagnoses'
- those people diagnosing with the DSM often change diagnoses or dispute diagnoses, and this can occur *both* because the client's actual behaviours *have* changed over time and because the diagnoses are not a good category system
- the apathy of institutions and individuals to actually look closely into the client's worlds; the professionals are often tightly constrained by how much time and effort they can put into contextual observations, especially outside the office (they often would like to, and I know some who 'secretly' do)

An example

As an example of seeing new connections once we dispense with the DSM-framed thinking, I was recently reading a lot of first-hand experiencers' accounts of their distress (as we all should do), as well as talking to people directly (as research). On one particular afternoon, I read an account of *a strong panic attack* first, then another person's account of *a strong visual hallucination,* and then another account of *hearing voices with a strong and critical voice* outside them for the first time.

These accounts were so similar in many, many ways, and probably were each *functioning* as desperate and exaggerated ways of getting some effect out of their bad life situations and making life change for them, even if just a little. It occurred to me: what really is the difference here?

- the person describing their panic attack felt the world closing in on them. They could not move (and they were in a car). They had multiple bad thoughts 'going through their head', and these were very anxiety provoking, so they felt paralyzed. They could not move from their car seat and crouched, scared.
- the person describing their hallucination also felt a vision closing in on them. Instead of bad anxiety thoughts 'in their head' (as for the panic attack), they saw a scary 'being' come through the wall and the 'being' was going to kill all the people around them. They crouched beneath a table and imagined they were screaming (even though they probably were not).
- the person hearing a voice for the first time also described the panic and fright at hearing a bad critical voice close to them but 'outside' yelling bad things at them. Again, the experience was one of their (bad) world finally closing in on them, so that something new and exceptional (and scary) was happening now. They too, could not escape this experience which made it worse.

All three experienced (1) a strong and powerful force upsetting their world totally, (2) which was not under their control at all, (3) which immobilized them, and (4) made them very scared. One person saw a very shocking hallucination; one heard multiple and insistent voices constantly repeating anxiety talk, saying negative and shocking things (as their own voice and anxious thoughts occurring 'inside their head'); and one had the same experience, but hearing that voice as coming from close but outside and independent of them. One happened to be a bad insistent *visual event*, one bad insistent *thoughts* (said to be their own internal voice), and the other a bad insistent *outside voice*.

Are these so different? But if we look in the DSM (as I then did) and interpret these as 'symptoms' of 'mental disorders', the DSM shows *no connection* between them except for the voice hearing and the hallucination—the panic attack is not even listed as comorbid or in differential diagnosis with the other two.

Now I might be wrong about this connection ('more research needed'), but my point here is that by putting all these behaviours or events into the DSM category system, an artificial and poorly constructed system at that (Caplan, 1995; Davies, 2014), *we do not even look for* new connections and possibilities. We are probably missing a lot that is going on that only first-hand experiencers might tell us, whether or not this particular connection I noticed holds up in other individual cases.

Summary of contextual model of 'mental health' (effects of being under stress or living in bad life situations which restrict any alternative behaviours)

In this chapter I have tried to take Frankl's well-known quote seriously—that the 'mental health' behaviours are 'abnormal' only because they are reactions from living in 'abnormal' situations. This has led to detailed discussions of what those 'abnormal' behaviours are, what those 'abnormal' situations are, and how those situations can shape the 'mental health' behaviours which are found, and which are distressful.

In doing this, we have seen that trying to live in bad life situations shapes *many* behaviours and strategies, not just those listed as 'mental health' behaviours. These include delinquent and criminal behaviours and life strategies of escape, exiting, and running away behaviours and strategies, and finding alternative lifestyles. It was suggested that all those involved in any of these behaviours who have expertise in preventing or changing the bad life situations (whether they are first-hand experiencers or professionals), should work together more since they share experience of a similar pool of bad situations which shape any of these.

It was also found that each of these life strategies developed under particular contexts, most requiring specialized skills or available resources. Important for this book were four special contexts revolving around having life options restricted or tightly controlled, and which shape the 'mental health' behaviours. We then saw that there were more specific contexts for when some of the 'mental health' behaviours would be likely to appear.

Finally, once the notion of 'mental health' as a biological disease is gone, it was suggested that all people living in bad life situations would be *shaped into more than one* of the crime, escape, 'mental health', and alternative lifestyle strategies (Woodiwiss, 1950). Likewise, those being shaped in the specific 'mental health' contexts would also be *shaped into more than one* of the 'mental health' behaviours, at different times and for different periods. The reason that this diversity has been overlooked is due to the way the DSM has overshadowed other approaches, and that it rigidly focuses both observations and analysis of the so-called 'mental health' contexts and behaviours far too narrowly.

What can we learn for therapy and healing?

The story so far is somewhat general, but the basic procedures are there. We need to:

- fully listen to the person's stories of their lived experience (taking them seriously)
- observe and inquire about specific contexts which were in place, following Box 8.1
- observe and inquire about specific 'mental health' contexts which were in place, following Figure 8.3
- observe and inquire about the range of behaviours, looking for both 'non-mental health' behaviours (Figure 8.1) as well as multiple 'mental health' behaviours (Box 8.2), and do not limit your 'search' to a single one for use as a diagnosis
- observe and inquire about the contexts which made other solutions over time not possible (Figure 8.2)
- look for the 'ordinary' origins of the behaviours and discuss the functions of these with the person
- we will see later that we must be cautious of too much questioning or inquiry, however, since sometimes this becomes yet another restrictive context for the person (like interrogation), and since many times the person *cannot* put into words their experience (and music, art, etc. might help here)

References

Adler, P. A. & Adler, P. (2012). *Constructions of deviance: Social power, context, and interaction.* London: Wadsworth.

Agnew, R. (2005). *Why do criminals offend? A general theory of crime and delinquency.* London: Oxford University Press.

Allsop, K., Read, J., Corcoran, R., & Kinderman, P. (2019). Heterogeneity in psychiatric diagnostic classification. *Psychiatry Research*, 279, 15–22.

American Psychiatric Association. (2013). *The diagnostic and statistical manual of mental disorders* (5th Ed.). Washington: APA.

Belknap, J. (2007). *The invisible woman: Gender, crime, and justice.* London: Wadsworth.

Bentall, R. P. (2006). Madness explained: Why we must reject the Kraepelinian paradigm and replace it with a 'complaint-orientated' approach to understanding mental illness. *Medical Hypotheses, 66*, 220–233.

Bloomfield, M. A. P., Chang, T., Wood, M. J., *et al.* (2021). Psychological processes mediating the association between developmental trauma and specific psychotic symptoms in adults: A systematic review and meta-analysis. *World Psychiatry, 20*, 107–123.

Brill, D. (2008). *Goth culture: Gender, sexuality and style.* NY: Berg.

Caplan, P. J. (1995). *They say you're crazy: How the world's most powerful psychiatrists decide who's normal.* NY: Life Long.

Cohen, S. (Ed.). (1971). *Images of deviance.* London: Penguin.

Cohen, S., & Taylor, L. (1976). *Escape attempts: The theory and practice of resistance to everyday life.* London: Allen Lane.

Cullen, F. T., & Agnew, R. (Eds.) (2003). *Criminological theory: Past to present.* Los Angeles, CA: Roxbury.

Dahrendorf, R. (1979). *Life chances: Approaches to social and political theory.* Chicago, IL: University of Chicago Press.

Damousi, J. (1997). *Depraved and disorderly: Female convicts, sexuality and gender in colonial Australia.* London: Cambridge University Press.

Davies, J. (2014). *Cracked: Why psychiatry is doing more harm than good.* London: Icon Books.

Decker, S. H., & Van Winkle, B. (1996). *Life in the gang: Family, friends, and violence.* New York: Cambridge University Press.

DeNora, T. (2015). *Music asylums: Wellbeing through music in everyday life.* London: Routledge.

Eckert, P. (1989). *Jocks and burnouts: Social categories and identity in the High School.* NY: Teachers College Press.

Feinberg, L. (1996). *Transgender warriors: Making history from Joan of Arc to Dennis Rodman.* Boston: Beacon Press.

Frankl, V. E. (2006). *Man's search for meaning.* NY: Beacon Press.

Fromene, R., & Guerin, B. (2014). Talking to Australian Indigenous clients with borderline personality disorder labels: Finding the context behind the diagnosis. *Psychological Record, 64*, 569–579.

Glasper, I. (2006). *The day the country died: A history of Anarcho Punk 1980 to 1984.* London: Cherry Red Books.

Goodlad, L. M. E., & Bibby, M. (Eds.). (2007). *Goth: Undead subculture.* Durham: Duke University Press.

Guerin, B. (2016). *How to rethink human behavior: A practical guide to social contextual analysis.* London: Routledge.

Guerin, B. (2017). *How to rethink mental illness: The human contexts behind the labels.* London: Routledge.

Guerin, B. (2020a). *Turning mental health into social action.* London: Routledge.

Guerin, B. (2020b). *Turning psychology into social contextual analysis.* London: Routledge.

Guerin, B. (2020c). *Turning psychology into a social science.* London: Routledge.

Guerin, B., Leugi, G. B., & Thain, A. (2018). Attempting to overcome problems shared by both qualitative and quantitative methodologies: Two hybrid procedures to encourage diverse research. *The Australian Community Psychologist, 29*, 74–90.

Hacking, I. (1998). *Mad travellers: Reflections on the reality of transient mental illness.* London: University Press of Virginia.

Haley, J. (1973). *Uncommon therapy: The psychiatric techniques of Milton H. Erickson, M.D.* London: Norton.

Haley, J. (Ed.) (1985). *Conversations with Milton H. Erickson, M.D. Volume 1: Changing individuals.* NY: Triangle Press.

Hartman, S. (2019). *Wayward lives, beautiful experiments: Intimate histories of riotous black girls, troublesome women, and queer radicals.* NY: Norton.

Hewett, P. (2004). *Racovia: An early liberal religious community.* Providence, RI: Blackstone Editions.

Hewitt, K. (1997). *Mutilating the body: Identity in blood and ink.* Bowling Green, OH: Bowling Green University Popular Press.

James, W. (1958/1902). *The varieties of religious experience: A study in human nature.* New York: The New American Library.

Johnstone, L. (2014). *A straight talking introduction to psychiatric diagnosis.* London: PCCS Books.

Johnstone, L., Boyle, M., Cromby, J., Dillon, J., Harper, D., Kinderman, P., … Read, J. (2018). *The Power Threat Meaning Framework: Towards the identification of patterns in emotional distress, unusual experiences and troubled or troubling behaviour, as an alternative to functional psychiatric diagnosis.* Leicester, UK: British Psychological Society.

Kinderman, P. (2019). *A manifesto for mental health: Why we need a revolution in mental health care.* London: Palgrave Macmillan.

Malvaso, C. G., Delfabbro, P. H., & Day, A. (2016). Risk factors that influence the maltreatment-offending association: A systematic review of prospective and longitudinal studies. *Aggression and Violent Behavior, 31,* 1–15.

Matza, D. (1969). *Becoming deviant.* Englewood Cliffs, NJ: Prentice Hall.

Maylea, C. (2021). The end of social work. *British Journal of Social Work, 51,* 772–789.

Mayo, P. E. (1969). *The making of a criminal: A comparative study of two delinquency areas.* London: Weidenfeld and Nicolson.

Mills, C. W. (1959). *The sociological imagination.* Oxford: Oxford University Press.

Nordhoff, C. (1966/1875). *The communistic societies of the United States: From personal visit and observation.* New York: Dover.

Orwell, G. (1933). *Down and out in Paris and London.* London: Victor Gollancz.

Richards, S. (n.d.). *BrainyQuote.com.* Retrieved June 22, 2020, from BrainyQuote.com website.

Rose, A. M. (1962). A social-psychological theory of neurosis. In A. M. Rose (Ed.), *Human behavior and social processes: An interactionist approach* (pp. 537–549). Boston: Houghton Mifflin.

Rowe, P. (2018). *Heavy metal youth identities: Researching the musical empowerment of youth transitions and psychosocial wellbeing.* London: Emerald Publishing.

Rowe, P., & Guerin, B. (2018). Contextualizing the mental health of metal youth: A community for social protection, identity and musical empowerment. *Journal of Community Psychology, 46,* 1–13.

Sartwell, C. (2014). *How to escape: Magic, madness, beauty, and cynicism.* NY: Excelsior Editions.

Todorov, T. (1997). *Facing the extreme: Moral life in the concentration camps.* NY: Henry Holt.

Tolokonnikova, N. (2018). *Read & riot: A Pussy Riot guide to activism.* NY: HarperOne.

Truong, F. (2018). *Radicalized loyalties: Becoming Muslim in the west.* London: Polity.

Turnbull, C. M. (1973). *The mountain people.* London: Jonathan Cape.

Wacquant, L. (2008). *Urban outcasts: A comparative sociology of advanced marginality*. London: Polity.

Wardlow, H. (2006). *Wayward women: Sexuality and agency in a New Guinea society*. London: University of California Press,

Watkins, M., & Shulman, H. (2008). *Toward psychologies of liberation*. London: Palgrave Macmillan.

Watson, J. (2019). *Drop the disorder: Challenging the culture of psychiatric diagnosis*. London: PCCS Books.

Woodiwiss, J. C. (1950). *Mad or bad? Studies of criminal insanity or wilful wrongdoing*. London: Quality Press.

Wyatt-Brown, B. (1988). The mask of obedience: Male slave psychology in the old South. *American Historical Review*, 93, 1228–1252.

Yablonsky, L. (1962). *The violent gang*. London: Penguin.

9 How changing context can change action, talking, and thinking

Analysing collateral and legacy effects

In Chapter 8 we saw new ways of viewing or rethinking 'mental health', which treats the 'mental health' behaviours as just *those behaviours being shaped by bad life contexts which are usually restrictive of alternative behaviours*. This has been suggested many times by many people (Frankl, for example), but never followed through into the details, which is what I am doing here. What is important to follow for this book about therapies is that this also changes our very ideas about what treatments, therapy, and 'cures' are all about (Chapter 10).

Of course, people's bad life situations can change over time but that does not mean the problems are then all gone, nor that they should now just be able to "get over it!" A lot of therapy is with people who *have had* bad life situations to deal with and those situations are finished, maybe the bad life situations were when they were very young, but there are still major effects on their current behaviours, talking, thinking, and feelings. I will refer to these as *legacy* effects and try to show ways that they are shaped by life situations, not from some inner person 'holding onto' behaviours, thoughts, and feelings.

The main thinking is that the original threats, traumas, or bad life situations altered all the other contexts for the person, so that even when the original threat or bad situation has passed, their actions, talking, and thinking have already been shaped in other ways that now cause them suffering. This is what we will try and begin explicating in this Chapter (in the tables of suggestions, primarily).

This chapter is to orient readers as to different ways this can occur, so we do not just have to give up hope but might find ways forward with the person. When a bad situation stops, the shaped behaviours *do not automatically stop* (people cannot always just "get over it!"), nor is it that a bad situation *always* leads to problems (early bad events do not always lead to trauma and problems later in life).

So, we need to be aware that there are ways that these different paths can happen for people; but in this chapter, I want to start a new conversation on the way behaviours might keep going and ways in which no behaviours continue. More observation, talking, and research needs to be done on these issues I will put forward, and the tables will be suggestions only. We need to get beyond the binary that traumatic events will always cause problems later in life,

DOI: 10.4324/9781003300571-12

and that when a person is out of a bad situation that their problems will just stop. This use of a binary has led to some unhealthy discussions and practices in therapy.

And as always in this area (Chapter 1), if we cannot see why the person cannot just "Get over it" when their bad life situation has stopped or cannot see why a bad life event might not have had an effect, then these are once again attributed to a literary plethora of fictional 'inner' stories. And once again, the observations are good but when the contexts are not explored then 'internal' attributions are dragged in once again. I do not have all the answers below, of course, but I wish to start a more detailed contextual conversation and let research look for better contextual observations to lead us forward.

How changing contexts change actions, talking, thinking, and feeling

In the broadest possible sense, the contextual message is that to change someone's behaviours, you need to change their contexts, in ways shown in Box 9.1.

Box 9.1 Basic social contextual conception of changing behaviours

To change someone's behaviours:

- Change the contexts which are shaping the behaviours
- Arrange new contexts which can shape the sorts of behaviours they want instead
- Most important are the social and societal contexts of life, which mediate all the things we need
- Change the available opportunities afforded by any life contexts

Of course, such human 'contexts' are very complex and very difficult to observe and change (Guerin, 2016). They include societal, economic, patriarchal, and cultural contexts; not just the physical objects around us, and these are difficult to change. But we can use this framework to get a new view of what traditional talking therapies might be doing that works or not (how the *Hugging Trees* or *Watching the Stars* therapies might have worked by inadvertently changing people's contexts).

The other major initial change in thinking about therapies from a social contextual view is that contextually we would not expect to see any of the 'mental health' behaviours 'cured' in the way envisaged by medical models—like when an infection is cured by giving antibiotics. Instead of a 'cure', if we apply the broad ideas of Box 9.1, we need to be thinking that when the shaping contexts are changed, the 'mental health' behaviours *disappear*, become *irrelevant*, become *unnecessary, go into the background, fade away,* or *do not show up anymore*, instead of thinking that they will be 'cured' and then stop. *Box 9.2* shows some of these. This has been often said by those who have had 'mental health' behaviours, although most also say that the behaviours are still there (that is, they are still possible when in the appropriate contexts) and are sometimes still useful or necessary. This aligns with the idea in Chapter 8 that these are ordinary behaviours gone wrong, so that they are still useful or necessary in some life contexts, and you would not want to completely 'unlearn' them or have them cease forever—just the extreme or exaggerated versions.

Box 9.2 Therapy is successful when the behaviours:

Medical models of 'mental health'	Contextual models of 'mental health'
stop	disappear
are 'cured'	become irrelevant
are blocked	become unnecessary
are corrected	go into the background
are fixed	fade away
'relapse' means the behaviours were not properly 'cured'	do not show up anymore (unless needed)
	can still be used in appropriate contexts
	'relapse' means the original contexts have returned

To get a feel for what this difference means, think about a skill you have which you do not use all the time. It could be a musical skill such as playing piano, guitar or oboe, it could be a thinking skill such as calculating multiplications or listing the capital cities of different countries, or it could be a skill like playing a card game or reciting the words of a Christmas carol. I picked these skills because they usually happen in life only in certain contexts: when there is a piano or guitar in front of us, when in a trivial game to name capital cities, or when on holiday once a year and the family plays card games. For many people, these are not behaviours that occur out of a specific context. You do not normally just start thinking about capital cities of the world or start air-playing an oboe.

But when you are *not* doing these behaviours, we would *not* say that you are cured or that the behaviours have been fixed, stopped or erased. And as soon as you are given the context (someone deals the cards, you sit down in front of a piano) and the behaviours return, albeit with a little warm-up, and we would not call this a 'relapse'. But our common 'mentalistic' talk (Chapter 1) 'explains' that you 'store' these behaviours in a memory and 'you' retrieve them, but this makes it seem as though you could 'remember' without any context at all, and also that you control the 'remembering' rather than the context controlling the 'remembering'. More simply, these behaviours are shaped by the contexts in which they were learned and reappear in those contexts.

I will give another example of this tricky but vital point, one that uses language and thinking as the relevant behaviours, which is more like most of the 'mental health' behaviours'. I recently met up, through some friends, a couple of people I went to high school with (hundreds of years ago!) and whom I had not seen since that time. Over a meal, I started 'remembering' things and saying things from that period, a long time ago in my case. These were thoughts, jokes, stories, people and names, events, and even emotions (I had a crush on one back then), that I had *never* thought about since. Outside of that reunion context, these language behaviours would never have occurred at all.

As mentioned above, calling this 'remembering' puts the agency onto a fictitious 'internal' person who 'decides' to remember, and it is also inaccurate or misleading to say that the context 'triggers' the language behaviours, since there are no specific parts that act like a trigger. And as always for 'internal' and 'mentalistic' explanations, you can also then be blamed for not remembering and have to take responsibility (we normally blame it in turn on our brain malfunctioning!). Other researchers talk in a better way by saying that the context '*engenders*' the behaviours, '*occasions*' the behaviours, or simply 'increases the probability' of the behaviours.

Basically, *put the context back and the behaviours occur again; the more specific the contexts, the more specific the behaviours.* This is also the approach of 'cognitive interviewing' used by police and others, although those methods *talk* to the person about contexts rather than put them actually back into that context (e. g., Collins, 2014). Given 'cognitive' means 'language use' (Guerin, 2020), cognitive interviewing uses language to give people the contexts in a verbal form rather than the real context itself. The real context would be preferable but not always possible, especially in police interviewing, so you are stuck with 'giving' context through using language.

The point of this is to realize that therapy and more generally *how to assist in changing the behaviours shaped from living in bad life situations* ultimately means *changing those bad life situations for the person* or else changing or adding other contexts so the bad situations lose their influence (Premack's principle). We will see below that even when bad situations have changed those behaviours and other unhelpful collateral behaviours can still continue, we will analyze these in the same way. This also makes us mindful of a point brought out in Chapter 2, that if a therapist assists a person in changing their behaviours (CBT for example) within a 'therapy' context, and the person then goes back to their usual bad life situation, the change will not be maintained most likely, although we saw in Chapter 5 how most current therapies have some components that assist the person even in such a case.

Some common collateral effects of bad life situations, which can leave a legacy even after they stop

In Chapter 8 we saw some broad strategic behaviours which are shaped by having to live in bad life situations: crime and delinquency, drugs and distractions, talking your way out of trouble, running away and other forms of exiting, using bullying or violence, or setting up a new life somewhere else (Figure 8.1). If these are not possible and life and opportunities are further restricted, then 'normal' behaviours can be shaped to be exaggerated because these give the impression that they have some immediate effects to bring about change but which usually do not (Figures 8.3 and 8.4). The latter are what have been called 'mental health' behaviours.

We are just beginning to explore all this, and other very useful approaches are given in the Power Threat Meaning Framework (Johnstone & Boyle, 2018), especially Chapter 4 on some common social contexts and their legacies, and Chapter 6 on some 'provisional general patterns' (also Boyle & Johnstone, 2020). If you can translate all the 'internal' metaphors to find the *external* threats that are present and shaping behaviour, then it is also worth going through the 29 'schemas' from schema therapy as well (Young, Klosko, & Weishaar, 2003, Table 1.1).

But none of these are fixed and they do not form a new replacement DSM category system. Every individual will be idiosyncratic because their contexts are idiosyncratic. But the patterns can be useful to sensitize you to new and better observations. So trust your observations more than what you read in these places or in my tables, and remember that certainty will only come from detailed case studies which explore the social contextual and discursive histories of those persons. There are many overlaps in these suggestions, which is encouraging, but individuals will not quite fit either, as idiosyncratic features of their lives come into play. The real goal of this chapter and the tables is to *sensitize* the reader to observe new idiosyncrasies for each new person with their unique life contexts.

Figure 9.1 tries to give a preliminary overview of where we have got to so far. Living in bad life situations shapes a lot of different behaviours. If the life options are restricted, then we begin to see behaviours shaped which we have been calling 'mental health' behaviours (although they are neither 'mental' nor to do with health directly). All the behaviours which are shaped from bad life situations also have collateral effects which can make matters worse. And even when the bad life situations can be stopped there are usually some legacy behaviours remaining which still cause suffering.

For the rest of this chapter, therefore, there are only *some suggestions of common patterns* you might find when doing social contextual analyses of people who have lived in bad life situations, to find out and observe the many collateral and legacy effects such living can produce.

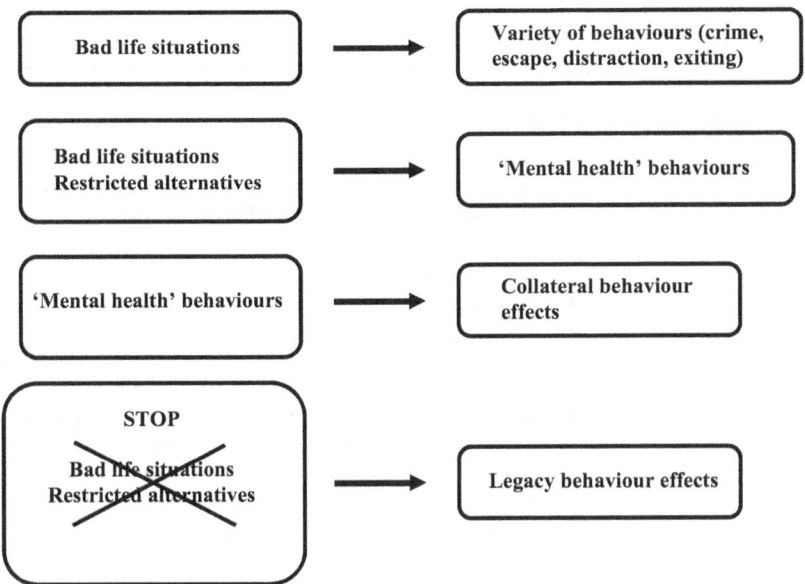

Figure 9.1 The effects of bad life situations and collateral and legacy effects

Common collateral effects of bad contexts

Another way to expand how we observe and ask about the changes in life context strategies is to consider some common collateral effects of one change leading to another. Nothing make these absolute and exceptions will always be found since life contexts are very idiosyncratic and something appearing in one person's life contexts will not be affecting another's. They are given here only to help sensitize you to some possible ways that the external and potentially observable changes in a person's contexts from sudden or chronic bad life situations leads to new behaviours (which might look like they appear from nowhere to casual observers and to those who make internal attributions).

Table 9.1 shows a number of collateral effects and contexts from the main bad life situations. That is, when trying to live in these situations, the table lists other possibilities which might co-occur and can be checked by observations and listening to your clients.

For example, if you live amidst a lot of violence then this models violence, so you and others are more likely to use it in future, so it becomes locked in future relationships. It becomes difficult for anyone to break out unless they exit or use other strategies. Other parts of society (school, bureaucracy, government) do not allow the use of violence to get one's way, so the person runs into trouble rapidly. Except within the violence-prone groups themselves (which can be violence-competitive), violence is also kept secret, so this

Table 9.1 Collateral effects of trying to live in various bad life situations (not mutually exclusive)

People trying to live in these bad life situations (or with these threats)	Possible collateral effects (can be observed but are pathologized and internalized by the medical models and the DSM)
Situations of violence	• Shapes people into the further uses of violence and bullying as solutions; modelling is available • Becomes locked in as further violence is usually a consequence of violence • Shapes escape and avoidance strategies in life • Makes difficulties when interacting with bureaucracies and 'societal controls' because violence is not tolerated as a social strategy • If talking is effective, then it shapes 'talking your way out' and manipulative uses of language • Increases secrecy, therefore, increases thinking over talking and increases uses of lying • Increases secrecy, and therefore makes it difficult to opt out or pursue new life strategies
Situations of delinquency and crime	• Increases secrecy, therefore increases thinking over talking and increases uses of lying • Increases secrecy, and therefore makes it difficult to opt out or pursue new life strategies • Becomes locked in • Shapes other escape and avoidance strategies in life • Likely to include situations of violence
Situations in which drug use is common	• Can prevent trying other solutions to bad situations • Becomes a solution to *any* bad situation • Becomes locked in, with many risks from long-term use • Increases confusion, and therefore makes it difficult to opt out or create new life strategies • In some cases, economic resources are needed, which leads to other issues and collateral contexts • Need for secrecy if illegal or taken to excess, so some social relationships will become altered, and some potentially supportive social relationships lost • It can calm down and reduce symptoms and help, if people are supported and guided to do other things
Situations of poverty	• In modern society lack of money restricts almost all access and opportunities for all resources • In modern society lack of money restricts almost all access and opportunities for social relationship building • Difficult to find other realistic solutions for bad situations with no money • Also restricts the 'power' for your discourses to have any effect within social relationships since resources are needed for language to function (Table 9.3) • Shapes behaviours, talking and thinking which appear unusual because most people have these shaped by money to align with marketing, commercialism, etc.

People trying to live in these bad life situations (or with these threats)	*Possible collateral effects (can be observed but are pathologized and internalized by the medical models and the DSM)*
Situations in which the person is forced to "put up with" their life situation	• Increases secrecy, therefore increases thinking over talking and increases uses of lying • Increases secrecy, and therefore makes it difficult to opt out or pursue new life strategies • Needs distractions and some forms of having effects, which can lead to further complications • Does allow time to gradually shape new strategies for changing life situations
Situations which are highly restrictive of alternative behaviours or highly oppressive (tight familial or societal control, bureaucratic, and legal systems)	• Lack of opportunities, whether through poverty, oppressive control, or disabilities, means that most other life contexts are changed even though not the person's fault • Becomes locked in • Normal behaviours can become exaggerated ('mental health' behaviours) if it appears that they can possibly change the life situation
Situations in which effective uses of language are broken (due to broken social relationships)	• See Table 9.3
Situations in which escape strategies have unintended effects (drugs, either recreational or psychiatric, entertainment of all sorts)	• Many of the escape or exiting responses to sudden or chronic bad life situations can be useful in the short term, especially when they give a calm and unhurried opportunity to find better long-term strategies • Many can themselves have bad long-term effects and constitute their own bad life situations • Psychiatric drugs fall into this category as they can initially produce some calm, which, if acted upon can help facilitate longer term changes to contexts, but the drugs themselves have bad side-effects if used for longer, which lead to collateral and legacy effects
Situations of colonization and oppressed Indigenous communities	• Most of the threats or bad life situations in this table apply (poverty, control, etc.) • Whole groups and communities undergo these bad life situations together and simultaneously which can lead to even more complex collateral effects (which is why these effects are real but not simple to analyze: Danieli, 1998; Kirmayer, Gone, & Moses, 2014; Maxwell, 2014; Mohatt, Thompson, Thai, & Tebes, 2014; Paradies, 2016) • Some effects of undergoing this together can be used advantageously • But undergoing collectively can also mean that conflict and disruptions can inadvertently occur within the group • The sources which shape colonized behaviours are usually opaque because they are diffused across interactions with many strangers in society and media, so attributions to self are common

People trying to live in these bad life situations (or with these threats)	Possible collateral effects (can be observed but are pathologized and internalized by the medical models and the DSM)
Situations of patriarchy, especially being female	• Gives power to others since they have privileges
	• The sources which shape gendered behaviours are usually opaque because they are diffused across interactions with many strangers in society and media, so attributions to self are common ("I like wearing makeup", "I would never wear makeup!")
	• Restricts behaviour and talking for many and narrows range of behaviours 'allowed', leading to collateral effects for restricted opportunities (see above) and lack of effects for talking and discourses (see Table 9.3)
	• In almost all cases such restrictions are more thorough and damaging for females than males
Situations of short-term traumatic events of all sorts with few outwardly noticeable effects (rape, assault, etc.)	• Needs new discourse, stories and self-narratives to portray world even within established social relationships
	• Can lead to avoiding social relationships if difficult to talk about
	• Shapes secrecy and covering up about the events, especially when stigma prevails (common)
	• Often there are physical injuries so there are new medical contexts to deal with, which can also alter previous social relationships or need secrecy strategies
	• Sometimes economic contexts are changed, and so resources are changed, which in turn change social relationships
Situations of sudden exposure to bad life situations (accidents, abuse, assault, loss of job)	• Difficulties having to talk about, explain and avoid being blamed
	• These difficulties mean that many or most social relationships are likely to be avoided or changed
	• People around will not understand living through such sudden and unexpected events since they are not common, so social relationships avoided even more
	• The effects of quick and hurried life strategies to deal with the sudden situation can go wrong immediately or in the longer term since they are not thought out well
	• Such hurried changes might be difficult to reverse later
	• Changing social relationships can also later mean changing economic exchanges
	• Sudden traumatic events are often in a very specific context and do not commonly reappear, so not only has the person no prior experience in how to respond (bad), but the same context is unlikely to reappear quickly so they can carry on regardless (good) if it were not for the other effects above of sudden bad life events

People trying to live in these bad life situations (or with these threats)	*Possible collateral effects (can be observed but are pathologized and internalized by the medical models and the DSM)*
Situations of long-term or chronic traumatic events or abuse of all sorts (physical, sexual, power, control)	• Increases some secrecy over a long time, therefore increases thinking over talking, and increases uses of lying • 'Disassociated' stories and self-narratives gradually used to portray world; that is, different stories for different social relationships • Social relationships become contradictory and compartmentalized • Thinking and talk become contradictory and compartmentalized • Avoidance of social relationships to avoid stories • Long term means more difficult to change, becomes locked in • Controlling social relationships will change most other life contexts • Being chronic, any strategies can become further embedded in the conflicts and make it more difficult to exit • There is more time for other bad effects to commence • It can lead to other consequences which are negative or make it difficult to exit later • There are difficulties maintaining face after an extended period which can lead to social relationship withdrawals • There are difficulties maintaining stories about yourself after an extended period • There are difficulties building new face or self-presentation after an extended period of being in a chronic bad life situation unless you find brand new social relationships • There are difficulties building new stories about yourself after an extended period unless you find brand new social relationships • Other people now rely on, and have built their own strategies around, that person's extended context, that is, other people now rely on them *not* changing • Environments change naturally but someone who has been in a chronic bad life situation might not be able to deal with this and make new changes in 'normal' ways
Situations in which oppressive and violent control taken over by individuals or groups	• Social relationships become contradictory and compartmentalized • Controlling social relationships will change most other life contexts • Usually outside social relationships are blocked • 'Disassociated' stories and self-narratives gradually used to portray world; it is still possible to talk to people outside the controlling relationship

People trying to live in these bad life situations (or with these threats)	*Possible collateral effects (can be observed but are pathologized and internalized by the medical models and the DSM)*
Situations in which 'benevolent' control taken over by individuals or groups	• The majority of people trying to help those in bad life situations are well-meaning but often not effective; this means that further withdrawals from social relationships are likely through escape or avoidance strategies, and then all the other effects that go with such withdrawals
Situations of exclusion or discrimination from social relationships	• Resources and other social connections coming through those relationships are now impossible • Requires finding alternative behaviours
Situations of being stigmatized for the exaggerated collateral behaviours which have been shaped by other contexts	• Being shaped into exaggerated 'normal' behaviours can lead others to stigmatize and avoid the person, thereby damaging social relationships • There might not be any obvious stigmatizing, but people might be reluctant to enter into social relationships when the person seems to have some exaggerated 'normal' behaviours • Some people strategize these behaviours to make them interesting or exciting to others, thereby making change more difficult since change might mean losing these social relationships
Situations of having disabilities and less flexible behaviour repertoires	• Restricts opportunities • Restricts social relationships • Many contextual restrictions which can probably be avoided but might need social support

discourages social relationships and leads to talking not being voiced (becomes thinking) except with aficionados. So even if violence is not done or talked about outside of the habitual groups and social relationships, there will still be a lot of violence-based thinking. Finally, unless you are successful at bullying and violence, then you will be oppressed by those in your groups who are good. All the above collateral contexts make this bad life situation even worse.

To take another example (and these should be expanded as you talk to new people about their very individual lives), short traumatic events like a car accident, rape, or a violent attack are bad. But on top of this there are a lot of collateral contextual changes which you need to learn from your talking to people in distress. Unless the traumatic event can be kept secret (which is often difficult), new stories about yourself and your life need to be trialled and experimented within your existing social relationships. You might need to change your beliefs or stories to deal with other people's comments and thoughts (even when well-intentioned). Sometimes the effects are injurious and medical systems and bureaucracies need to be negotiated at a time when this is least desired, and this will require further changes to your normal previous social relationships. All the above can also change your economic contexts, which will require major changes to your resourcing and social relationships. Often it is easier to just drop previous social relationships since there is so much discourse that needs to be changed and protected during conversations.

None of the above or Table 9.1 is prescriptive or categorical. Every person will be different depending upon their previous social relationships and resources. Once again, specific and idiosyncratic contextual observations and listening will be needed.

A final point to learn from this, which will become an important part of Chapter 11, is that for each of these bad situations there will be people with a lot of personal experience, whether first or second hand. They will know more of the nuances and collateral intricacies than my tables provide. Someone who does not have experience will be guessing and using generalities. So part of the solution for reimagining therapy is to make integrated use of other people for whom these tables are already well-known through experience and who know a lot more strategies and possible collateral effects than I have presented.

Some common behaviour patterns of legacy effects

Once the broad patterns of collateral contextual changes are understood we can discern both further collateral changes to people's lives and also the legacy effects so that when the immediate bad situations or threat stops, the shaped behaviours continue. Table 9.2 gives some examples to begin your explorations with individuals. These are not authoritative, just ways of sensitizing you to discern the patterns and others not covered in the tables.

As an example, many bad life situations or threats lead to conditions requiring secrecy. Having to maintain some secrecy leads in turn to many other collateral contextual changes in life, including more of the talking not being said out loud and hence increases in what is called thinking or rumination. Once discourses become thought rather than being said, then there are many other changes, including less consequation and hence those thought discourses become less likely to ever change or be modified (Table 7.2). This in turn can lead to excessive overthinking in some cases, and more extreme, abstract and generalized views in other cases. This also means that even if the main life bad situations or threats clear up these unconsequated thoughts are likely to continue as legacy effects. That is, the situations that shaped excessive or extreme discourses (as thinking) might cease but the thinking pattern remains (discourses not said out loud).

Some common behaviour patterns when discursive communities are disrupted or broken

The final table looks at the more specific bad life situations through which social and societal relationships become so disrupted that language ceases to

Table 9.2 Potential collateral and legacy effects of having lived in a bad life situation

Common collateral effects of bad situations which might linger	Further possible collateral and legacy effects
Social relationships are changed	• There are numerous ways that almost any effects of bad life situations also change a person's social relationships from what they were • Changing social relationships can also change economic and other resource contexts in turn; changing social relationships can also change current and future 'opportunity contexts' further limiting the person's life and chances of changing • Changes in social relationships are legacy effects in that if the bad situations stop, the original social relationships are unlikely to go back to what they were • Changes in social relationships also stop or change discursive relationships, that is, what can be done with words, and new discursive relationships are needed (e.g., finding new stories and ways of getting directives obeyed)
Increases use of secrecy strategies	• Most bad life situations, whether sudden or chronic lead to secrecy strategies for a multitude of reasons. • As a form of escape or exiting, secrecy can help in some ways but also then prevent better change strategies from occurring • Such strategies range from locking oneself away ('depressive' behaviours) to lying and deceit as strategic responses to bad events • Secrecy also means that thinking becomes more frequent as things once said out loud no longer are said • In turn, then, not saying things out loud has a collateral problem that language and discourses do not get consequated and so are less likely to change, so talking patterns (now thinking patterns) become incessant and recurring • This can be seen in anxiety (planning discourses gone wrong), rumination, and most of the 'thinking disorder' behaviours that are observed. • With secrecy strategies, stories and other discourses get compartmentalized into separate groups and so dissociation phenomena will occur
Increases uses of language where discursive communities are still functional	• When the response to bad life situations involves using language to escape or talk your way out, then such discourses can become inflexible to future changing circumstances • Using language in this way also leads to exaggerated 'planning' of language for any contingencies which might arise, that is, anxiety and rumination behaviours either out loud or as thinking • Using language in this way can lead to over-strong beliefs and opinions and 'fixed ideas' (Janet). • Also Table 9.3

Common collateral effects of bad situations which might linger	*Further possible collateral and legacy effects*
Increases the (emotional) behaviours done when there are no words for the bad life situations (through societal effects, social relationship contexts frequently, other hidden contexts shaping, complex situations)	• Many of the bad life situations cannot be put into words easily for a variety of reasons so many 'emotional' behaviours • People will further avoid talking and avoid social relationships if what has happened to them cannot be put into words • And avoid situations in which questions are asked, including therapy and professionals doing their job • They will use a lot of abstract emotional discourses • Emotional behaviours become common and exaggerated
Modelling from what happened and what has been observed	• The behaviours experienced or witnessed during bad life situations can modelled and repeated leading to further complications • Violence and abuse are often examples but cannot always be easily observed • Ways of using language can also be modelled
Collateral effects of poor health	• Sudden or chronic bad life situations, and the collateral effects being outlined here, also impact of physical health • living with poor physical health itself constitutes a further bad life situation with all that is required to deal with this
Dissatisfaction with mental health services and terminology.	• Given the difficulties arising from the medical model and its derived treatments, many of those with either sudden or chronic bad life situations have a difficult time within the 'mental health' services, and this can itself constitute another bad life situation that needs to be dealt with • This is especially apparent with forced admissions and forced treatments
Effects of seeing hypocrisies and being aware of contextual anomalies that other are not aware of	• With all the problems associated with either sudden or chronic bad life situations, and the lack of clear support, many of those develop a general mistrust of social relationships • Development of a special distrust of those in power and professional positions (even if well-intentioned) • They more readily notice the real hypocrisies in normal and professional life, which is useful to have realistic view of life, but can also lead to reducing the opportunities and fruitful social relationships which could be available otherwise.
Compartmentalization effects	• One change in modern life is that we have fragmented social relationships, in the sense that our different social relationships often have little or no contacts between them • This means that living in sudden or chronic bad life situations of all sorts can be easily kept secret from many of your social relationships, so they never know • This has a collateral effect that useful support might be missed because of this

Common collateral effects of bad situations which might linger	Further possible collateral and legacy effects
Leakages across contexts	• We have seen many examples of how problems in one life context 'leak' across to affect other life contexts • This is why examining all intersectionalities is so important, and a good knowledge of societal intersectionalities essential • The most common example is a bad life context (perhaps bullying and discrimination) leading to withdrawal from social relationships which reduces opportunities in life, which might be useful, and which leads to bad life economic contexts (in the broadest sense of resources)

have the normal effects such as getting people to do things, getting people to respond, or having humour and stories appreciated to form and maintain social relationships. These are life situations in which *any* talking might be neglected, opposed, ridiculed, or otherwise punished.

So, Table 9.3 has some *common ways* that people behave when their language no longer has effects. When people cannot get reactions and effects from using language, what do they do? Over a short time, or over a long time? Some suggestions only for you to build on.

Some of this can also be seen in persons with poor language abilities (for whatever reason) when they cannot get things done through other people by using words. When under stress and pressure, those with intellectual disabilities often become 'aggressive', gesticulate and flail, turn away, show a range of 'emotional' behaviours, or withdrawal from all social engagement.

Putting this all together

The tables are meant to begin finding ways to discern how real-life contexts shape the behaviours that have been called 'mental health' behaviours and attributed to hidden 'inside' workings of various sorts (Chapter 1). This is only a beginning, and the point is to become sensitized so you can discern the idiosyncratic life patterns of individuals, since any generic pattern will not always hold. The patterns are very complex and idiosyncratic (e. g., Farge & Foucault, 2016).

A good way to become sensitized to all the responses is to talk with people who have lived through this. From them, if you listen and question about observations rather than talk abstractions, you can develop a social contextual history and an idea of their discursive history (Chapter 10). Another way to become sensitized to these strategic and contextual patterns is to read first-hand accounts and then second-hand accounts, some of which are listed in Box 9.3.

Table 9.3 Some common ways that people behave when their language no longer has effects

Common collateral effects when discursive communities are not functioning, and language no longer has its usual effects	Further possible collateral and legacy effects
Using physical force	• When language is broken, and no effects are forthcoming by using words, physical means are often the first result • This can mean more touching or more bullying (physical), and everything in between • This can lead to further problems, of course, not directly related to what is breaking the language in the first place
Talking is exaggerated	• When language is broken, or beginning to snap, the result is often to exaggerate parts of talking or writing, as we have all learned that doing any of these increases the chances that our language will have some sort of effect • this can be exaggerated volume (loud or soft), word excesses, riskiness of the words (swear words or horror that get an effect), or the content of the talking or writing • You can even observe cases where grammar is perfected and (over) used, since we have learned that better grammar makes language more likely to work with many listeners
Talking reduces and thinking increases, with concomitant effects	• See Table 7.2 • Our words and discourses (as thought) will become shorter and pithy, ungrammatical, leave out room for turn-taking and repartee, with reduced facial and gestural affect shown ('negative symptoms') • More likely to have discourses (not out loud) which become about worse things than you would ever have said out loud, including cruder, more violent or aggressive, and ruder • Because 'thought' discourses are not consequated, a person's discourses will become less flexible to future changing circumstances; that is, their discourses ('thinking') becomes rigid and extreme • Likewise, any overuse of planning discourses becomes anxieties and ruminations, which again, because they are not consequated, become more difficult to change even with changes in the bad situations
Stories and 'self' get changed in unusual ways, hence also 'personality' and compartmentalization (dissociation) between different versions of stories	• When a person's stories, explanations and justifications become primarily thought only, they can become changed and exaggerated in ways that are unusual (delusions, obsessions, fixed ideas, etc.) • Because these are also not consequated by discursive communities, there can be several versions of the same discourses and show the range of dissociation phenomena

Common collateral effects when discursive communities are not functioning, and language no longer has its usual effects	*Further possible collateral and legacy effects*
Using those behaviours we do when language does not work—the ones we call 'emotional'	• In a contextual sense, emotional behaviours are those which appear (opportunistically) when words do not function, so more emotional behaviours will occur when language ceases to function in discursive communities • The exact behaviour is not necessarily related to the issues that have stopped the language exchanges from working; they can be just behaviours which happen to be available, common, easy, or resource-low
Using language more on strangers	• Many of the issues with broken language in life arise from significant others (family and friends) no longer responding to the person's language with any effects • A common response to this is to talk more with strangers, since strangers will usually allow small amounts of responding without money • This can lead to inappropriate attempts to get an effect from strangers with language • This can lead to a constant string of new strangers being approached
Doing things ourselves	• Another response to language not working is to do more of the things in life ourselves rather than relying on language to affect other people to do things • This can also lead to overachieving and excessive behaviours • As well, it can lead to stopping many behaviours altogether if they cannot be successfully done without help, leading to 'negative symptoms' and various behaviours currently labelled as 'depression' • People do not just spend time alone because they are sad, they can also do it because they cannot get things done with other people anymore and it is better to avoid than be punished
Stop behaving altogether	• Since so much of human behaviour is accomplished through using language, when this ceases to work people often give up trying • Withdrawal from social relationships of all types, and failure to engage in new social relationships ("What's the point?")
Pointing and poking a lot	• An increase in gesticulations is often observed • Similar increases can be seen when trying to get people who do not speak your language to do things through words

Common collateral effects when discursive communities are not functioning, and language no longer has its usual effects	Further possible collateral and legacy effects
Planning and organizing what we do	• One thing we all learn to do a lot with language is to talk through plans and life organization without saying this out loud. While this thinking/talking through does not control whether we do things or not (they are both actually shaped by our social relationships and exchanges), most people learn to do this and saying bits of it out loud gets a lot of positive effects from people (even whether or not we carry through with our plans). This is especially so for good neoliberal behaviour, to show that you are thinking ahead and planning • What this means is that when language gets messed up, even though our talking about plans has no effect on our social relationships anymore, the planning and thinking can continue unabated and consequated • This is one way to think about people who overthink, who report severe and constant anxieties, ruminations and intrusive thoughts, and who experience language conflicts when they both plan events in life and simultaneously talk through the likely bad outcomes of that same planning
Making friends	• When our social relationships break down (and hence our language does not work on those people anymore), we can be shaped to look for new friends • In bad life situations, however, this might become inappropriate, and people approached inappropriately who are thought to be suitable as friends, whether this is related to the age, lack of consent, not noticing their signs of displeasure, or other things
Laws	• We are constantly shaped that people follow laws and rules (words) even though what makes these actually work is out of our control • When language is not working this can lead to inappropriate uses of making and enforcing arbitrary rules that people around you 'should' follow, even though the normal hidden social exchanges which can make rules work are not there • This is observed as trying to impose general rules upon people who are close, as if just the words themselves will start effects occurring again
Making jokes	• We learn in life that making jokes can lead to positive effects, but again the hidden social exchanges and reciprocities are not usually obvious in everyday life (indeed, people believe that the words of jokes are what is funny; if the audience does not have the right relationship set up then jokes will not work, even what seem to be the funniest jokes or jokes you have seen 'work' elsewhere) • So, in the absence of your language working, jokes and being funny or silly can be tried (they have been shaped) but they are unlikely to work • This can once more lead to inappropriate attempts to get effects through being funny, amusing or silly in exaggerated ways

Common collateral effects when discursive communities are not functioning, and language no longer has its usual effects	*Further possible collateral and legacy effects*
Telling stories and gossip	• As kids we learn that to get more 'attention' (a range of effects) from telling stories if we exaggerate the story and add features ('sex drugs and rock and roll' or shock) which can increase listening and effects of storytelling • When language begins breaking down (social relationships, that is) and people no longer listen to or react to storytelling, then exaggerations are perhaps all that is left, and telling stories to strangers (see above) • From this, delusions, conspiracies and rumour-mongering are born
Social media	• If social relationships are weak and talking to people getting less and less effects, then social media have available all sorts of channels for doing so • Getting effects (hits) is what social media have been carefully made for in the first place (in order to get marketing) • As above, this might require constantly changing the strangers being engaged or exaggerating what is put on social media to get effects

Box 9.3 Examples of good first-hand and second-hand accounts of responding in bad life situations which have shaped 'mental health' and other behaviours, to help become sensitized to the complexities and nuances

First-hand accounts
Basset & Stickley, 2010; Broug, 2008; Bryant, 2020; Dee, 2009; Dorman, 2006; #Emerging Proud, 2019a, 2019b, 2019c; Factora-Borchers, 2014; Filer, 2019; Grant, Biley, & Walker, 2011; Harrison, 2014; inside out & associates australia and the Collaborative Book Project, 2019; Kaplan, 1964; Kavan, 1990; LeCroy & Holschuh, 2012; Ralls, 2021; Romme, Escher, Dillon, Corstens, & Morris, 2009; Schneider, 2010; Thomas, 2013; Watson, 2019, 2020; Xinran, 2002

Second-hand accounts and descriptive case-studies (For most of these you will need to remove the jargon and look for the basic observations)
Cameron & Magaret, 1951; Cleckley, 1964; Cohen, 1971; Cohen & Taylor, 1976; Costello, 1970; Damouse, 1997; Danieli, 1998; Decker & Van Winkle, 1996; Eckert, 1989; Figes, 1987; Glasper, 2006; Hacking, 1998; Hartman, 2009; Janet, 1902, 1907, 1925/1919; Johnstone & Boyle, 2018; Jung, 1960;

Longden, Corstens, Escher, & Romme, 2012; Maté, 2009; Mellon, 1998; Meyer, 1948; Milosz, 1968; Nordhoff, 1966/1875; Orwell, 1933; Prince, 1913; Qi, Palmier-Claus, Simpson, Varese, & Bentall, 2019; Reyes-Foster, 2009; Rogers, 2006; Rogers & Leydesdorff, 2004; Rokeach, 1984; Rowe, 2018; Sanchez, 2010; Sartwell, 2014; Schilder, 1950, 1976; Sullivan, 1973, 1974; Truong, 2018; Turnbull, 1973; Wardlow, 2006; Wyatt-Brown, 1988; Yablonsky, 1962

Two examples of living in bad life situations

Before leaving bad life situations and what they really look like, I will give two examples of real lives. These come from research case studies of people who at some point in their lives had been assigned a label of 'generalized anxiety disorder' (Beaton, 2014). There were a total of eight people and one of the main findings was that *they all were different*. In Figures 9.2 and 9.3 I show two examples of 'Brad' and 'Lucy'. Across all eight people the complexities looked similar to these even though their details were all different (despite them all getting the same 'diagnosis'!).

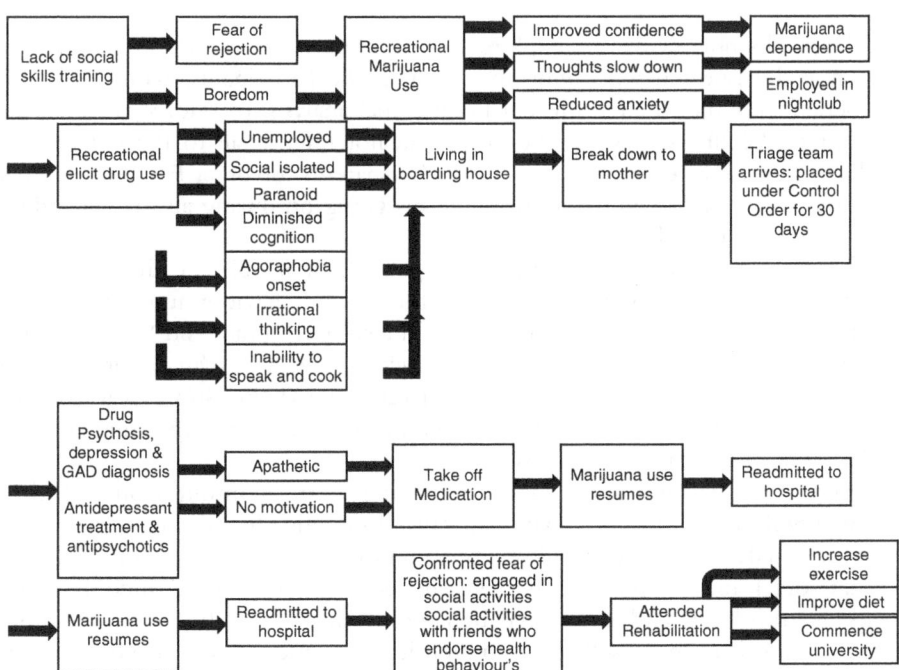

Figure 9.2 Real life pathway as reported by 'Brad' who had a 'Generalized Anxiety Disorder' label (reads from left to right and then continues below).

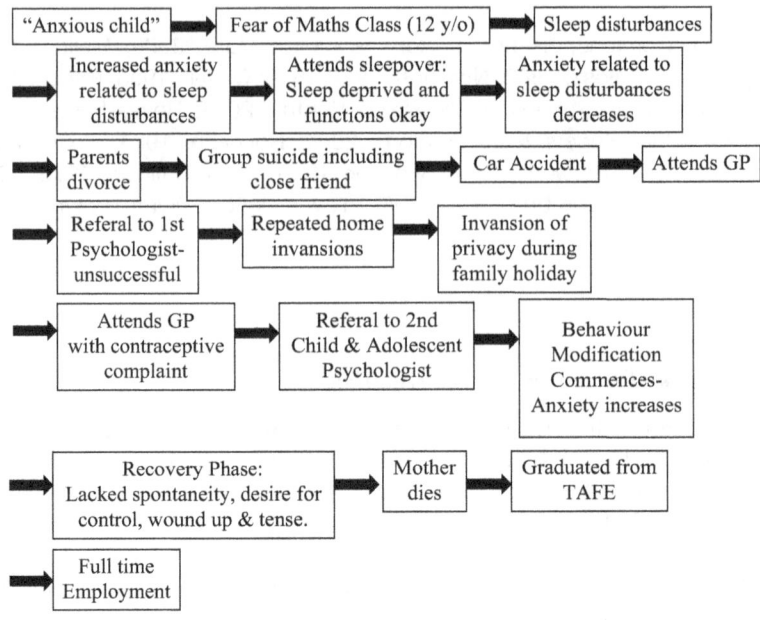

Figure 9.3 Real life pathway as reported by 'Lucy' who had a 'Generalized Anxiety Disorder' label.

These do not, however, explore the concrete contexts which are present because the research was trying to stay with the participants' words for their experiences, rather than a full social contextual analysis. In Lucy's pathway, for example, the first six events she noted did not refer at all to the contexts in which they occurred but the seventh is her parents' divorce. For a contextual analysis we would need to know what was going on during all this, including how her talking and thinking changed.

This demonstrates another important point: that people are frequently not aware of the contexts which are shaping their own behaviour and use the same 'internal' languages as professionals do, as indeed both 'Brad' and 'Lucy' did. Of even more special interest is that just as explaining a human event as being 'caused' by something internal leads to blaming the victim, so you can observe that people explaining their own behaviour as something originating 'internally' often blame themselves as well!

And the final important and interesting point coming from all this, which will be highlighted later in this book—is that doing social contextual analysis can by itself be 'therapeutic' in some ways. Finding out what social and societal forces have shaped your behaviour, including the talking, thinking, and emotional behaviours shaped by discursive communities, can lead by itself to therapeutic outcomes, even if you cannot completely change those forces (Chapter 10). Feminist therapists facilitate this by having clients join women's rights groups; Indigenous therapists encourage clients to go to decolonization workshops. Just *discerning* what has shaped your behaviours and your life, is extremely useful.

References

#Emerging Proud. (2019a). *Through NOTEs (non-ordinary transcendent experiences): Stories of hope & transformation.* Norwich, UK: Emerging Proud Press.

#Emerging Proud. (2019b). *Through suicide: Stories of hope & transformation.* Norwich, UK: Emerging Proud Press.

#Emerging Proud. (2019c). *Through trauma & abuse: Stories of hope & transformation.* Norwich, UK: Emerging Proud Press.

Basset, T. & Stickley, T. (2010). *Voice of experience: Narratives of mental health survivors.* London: Wiley-Blackwell.

Beaton, M. (2014). *Client perspectives of Generalised Anxiety Disorder.* Honours Thesis, University of South Australia.

Boyle, M., & Johnstone, L. (2020). *A straight talking introduction to the Power Threat Meaning Framework: An alternative to psychiatric diagnosis.* London: PCCS Books.

Broug, M. (2008). *Seventeen voices: Life and wisdom from inside 'mental illness'.* Adelaide: Wakefield Press.

Bryant, K. (2020). *Hysteria: A memoir of illness, strengths and women's stories throughout history.* Sydney: University of New South Wales Press.

Cameron, N. & Magaret, A. (1951). *Behavior pathology.* Boston: Houghton Mifflin.

Cleckley, H. (1964). *The mask of sanity: An attempt to clarify some issues about the so-called psychopathic personality.* Saint Louis: C.V.MosbyCompany.

Cohen, S. (Ed.). (1971). *Images of deviance.* London: Penguin.

Cohen, S., & Taylor, L. (1976). *Escape attempts: The theory and practice of resistance to everyday life.* London: Allen Lane.

Collins, D. (2014). *Cognitive interviewing practice.* London: Sage.

Costello, C. G. (Ed.). (1970). *Symptoms of psychopathology: A handbook.* NY: John Wiley.

Damouse, J. (1997). *Depraved and disorderly: Female convicts, sexuality and gender in colonial Australia.* London: Cambridge University Press.

Danieli, Y. (Ed.). (1998). *International handbook of multigenerational legacies of trauma.* NY: Plenum Press.

Decker, S. H., & Van Winkle, B. (1996). *Life in the gang: Family, friends, and violence.* New York: Cambridge University Press.

Dee, R. (2009). *Fractured: Living nine lives to escape my own abuse.* London: Hodder.

Dorman, P. (2006). *I cry for help: Autobiography/health, my true story detailing the aftermath of child abuse, trauma, stress, combat trauma, & post traumatic stress disorder.* NY: iUniverse.

Eckert, P. (1989). *Jocks and burnouts: Social categories and identity in the High School.* NY: Teachers College Press.

Factora-Borchers, L. (Ed.). (2014). *Dear sister: Letters from survivors of sexual abuse.* Edinburgh, Scotland: AK Press.

Farge, A., & Foucault, M. (2016). *Disorderly families: Infamous letters from the Bastille Archives.* London: University of Minnesota Press,

Figes, O. (1987). *The whisperers: Private life in Stalin's Russia.* London: Penguin Books.

Filer, N, (2019). *The heartland: Finding and losing schizophrenia.* London: Faber & Faber.

Glasper, I. (2006). *The day the country died: A history of Anarcho Punk 1980 to 1984.* London: Cherry Red Books.

Grant, A., Biley, F., & Walker, H. (2011). *Our encounters with madness*. London: PCCS Books.

Guerin, B. (2016). *How to rethink human behavior: A practical guide to social contextual analysis*. London: Routledge.

Guerin, B. (2020). *Turning psychology into social contextual analysis*. London: Routledge.

Hacking, I. (1998). *Mad travelers: Reflections on the reality of transient mental illness*. London: University Press of Virginia.

Harrison, K. (2014). *Pendulum: Poetic insights from a journey through mental illness*. Adelaide: Ginninderra Press.

Hartman, S. (2009). *Wayward lives, beautiful experiments: Intimate histories of riotous black girls, troublesome women, and queer radicals*. NY: W. W. Norton.

inside out & associates australia and the Collaborative Book Project. (2019). *Our own words: Reflections on living with mental distress and extreme states (and living without them)*. Sydney: inside out & associates australia

Janet, P. (1902). *The mental state of hystericals: A study of mental stigmata and mental accidents*. NY: G. P. Putnam's Sons.

Janet, P. (1907). *The major symptoms of hysteria*. London: Macmillan.

Janet, P. (1925/1919). *Psychological healing: A historical and clinical study*. London: George Allen & Unwin.

Johnstone, L. & Boyle, M. with Cromby, J., Dillon, J., Harper, D., Kinderman, P., Longden, E., Pilgrim, D. & Read, J. (2018). *The Power Threat Meaning Framework: Towards the identification of patterns in emotional distress, unusual experiences and troubled or troubling behaviour, as an alternative to functional psychiatric diagnosis*. Leicester: British Psychological Society.

Jung, C. G., (1960). *The psychogenesis of mental disease*. NY: Princeton University Press.

Kaplan, B. (1964). *The inner world of mental illness: A series of first person accounts of what it was like*. NY: Harpercollins.

Kavan, A. (1990). *My madness: The selected writings of Anna Kavan*. NY: Picador.

Kirmayer, L. J., Gone, J. P., & Moses, J. (2014). Rethinking historical trauma. *Transcultural Psychiatry*, 51, 299–319.

LeCroy, C. W., & Holschuh, J. (2012). *First person accounts of mental illness and recovery*. NY: John Wiley.

Longden, E., Corstens, D., Escher, S., & Romme, M. (2012). Voice hearing in a biographical context: A model for formulating the relationship between voices and life history. *Psychosis*, 4, 224–234.

Maté, G. (2009). *In the realm of hungry ghosts: Close encounters with addiction*. London: Vintage.

Maxwell, K. (2014). Historicizing historical trauma theory: Troubling the trans-generational transmission paradigm. *Transcultural Psychiatry*, 51, 407–435.

Mellon, J. (Ed.). (1998). *Bullwhip days: The slaves remember*. NY: Grove Press.

Meyer, A. (1948). *The commonsense psychiatry of Dr. Alfred Meyer: Fifty-two selected paper, with biographical narrative*. NY: McGraw-Hill.

Milosz, C. (1968). *The captive mind*: London: Penguin.

Mohatt, N. V., Thompson, A. B., Thai, N. D., & Tebes, J. K. (2014). Historical trauma as public narrative: A conceptual review of how history impacts present-day health. *Social Science & Medicine*, 106, 128–136.

Nordhoff, C. (1966/1875). *The communistic societies of the United States: From personal vat and observation*. New York: Dover.

Orwell, G. (1933). *Down and out in Paris and London*. London: Victor Gollancz.

Paradies, Y. (2016). Colonisation, racism and indigenous health. *Journal of Population Research*, 33, 83–96.

Prince, M. (1913). *The dissociation of a personality: A biographical study in abnormal psychology*. NY: Longmans, Green and Co.

Qi, R., Palmier-Claus, J., Simpson, J., Varese, F., & Bentall, R. (2019). Sexual minority status and symptoms of psychosis: The role of bullying, discrimination, social support, and drug use—Findings from the Adult Psychiatric Morbidity Survey 2007. *Psychology and Psychotherapy: Theory, Research and Practice*, 1–17.

Ralls, D. (2021). *Straightjacket to success*. London: Gnosis Publishing.

Reyes-Foster, B. M. (2019). *Psychiatric encounters: Madness and modernity in Yucatan, Mexico*. London: Rutgers University Press.

Rogers, K. L. (2006). *Life and death in the Delta: African American narratives of violence, resilience, and social change*. NY: Palgrave Macmillan.

Rogers, K. L., & Leydesdorff, S. (2004). *Trauma: Life stories of survivors*. London: Transaction Publishers.

Rokeach, M. (1984). *The three Christs of Ypsilanti: A psychological study*. NY: New York Review Books.

Romme, M., Escher, S., Dillon, J., Corstens, D., & Morris, M. (2009). *Living with voices: 50 stories of recovery*. London: PCCS Books.

Rowe, P. (2018). *Heavy metal youth identities: Researching the musical empowerment of youth transitions and psychosocial wellbeing*. London: Emerald Publishing.

Sanchez, A. C. (2010). *Fear and progress: Ordinary lives in Franco's Spain, 1939–1975*. London: Wiley-Blackwell.

Sartwell, C. (2014). *How to escape: Magic, madness, beauty, and cynicism*. NY: Excelsior Editions.

Schilder, P. (1950). *The image and the appearance of the human body: Studies in the constructive energies of the psyche*. NY: International Universities Press.

Schilder, P. (1976). *On psychoses*. NY: International Universities Press.

Schneider, B. (2010). *Hearing (our) voices: Participatory research in mental health*. Toronto: University of Toronto Press.

Sullivan, H. S. (1973). *Clinical studies in psychiatry*. NY: Norton.

Sullivan, H. S. (1974). *Schizophrenia as a suman process*. NY: Norton.

Thomas, M. E. (2013). *Confessions of a sociopath: A life spent hiding in plain sight*. London: Pan Books.

Truong, F. (2018). *Radicalized loyalties: Becoming Muslim in the west*. London: Polity.

Turnbull, C. M. (1973). *The mountain people*. London: Jonathan Cape.

Wardlow, H. (2006). *Wayward women: Sexuality and agency in a New Guinea society*. London: University of California Press.

Watson, J. (2019). *Drop the disorder: Challenging the culture of psychiatric diagnosis*. London: PCCS Books.

Watson, J. (Ed.). (2020). *We are the change-makers: Poems supporting Drop the Disorder*. London: PCCS Books.

Wyatt-Brown, B. (1988). The mask of obedience: Male slave psychology in the old South. *American Historical Review*, 93, 1228–1252.

Xinran (2002). *The good women of China: Hidden voices*. London: Vintage Books.

Yablonsky, L. (1962). *The violent gang*. London: Penguin.

Young, J. E., Klosko, J. S., & Weishaar, M. E. (2003). *Schema therapy: A practitioner's guide*. London: Guilford Press.

10 Summarizing the changes needed for 'therapy' after including social and societal contexts

It is time to summarize all that has been said so far and start talking about what we do next. This chapter will bring together all the themes and paint a broad picture of what needs to change with therapy while keeping what we can of current practices (but not the theories). Chapter 11 will look at the more specific details of what therapy might start doing differently.

It all depends on your thinking

As we have seen, starting in Chapter 1 but popping up throughout the rest of the chapters, so much of past and current therapy is shaped by *how you think about people and why they do what they do*. This is not just about developing your aims and goals of therapy (Chapter 3), or the procedures you use (Chapter 4), but also about what you consider normal approaches when engaging with another human being. This includes the whole idea of people seeing a *single* therapist, working from an office, keeping confidentiality, working under bureaucratic rules, being paid, having 'expert' status, and other hidden social and cultural assumptions (Box 1.1 and Chapter 2).

In particular, for this book, the whole historical thinking which I argued has defined psychology itself has been challenged by many; challenging that people have an 'inner' life—that there is someone in there looking out (Chapters 1 and 6). So much of the methods, practices, and procedures of all therapies rely on this assumption being true to make any sense, and when some of these practices do not work, stories are spun because that is easy when the 'science' is based on a fictional 'inner' life ("The person wasn't ready", "The person wasn't motivated", "The person had an inner dilemma preventing them").

Once this whole idea that there is another mysterious world called 'psychological' is gone, we do not lose everything that has been accomplished, but it opens up so much more. We mainly lose the talk, the theorizing, the marketing, and the feel-good stories, which have been wrapped around therapy for 100 years.

DOI: 10.4324/9781003300571-13

Analyze the contexts which shape our behaviours

We must therefore analyze the social, societal, economic, cultural, patriarchal, colonizing, and other life contexts which shape human behaviours if we are to make progress (Guerin, 2016). This applies not only to understanding people seeking help (Chapters 6, 7 and 8), but also to the notion of therapy itself as a practice shaped by imitating medical practices, from governmental need to control populations, and more recently from the bureaucratic control of large groups of strangers living together and having inevitable conflicts (Chapter 2, Guerin, 2020). This shift also changes our understanding of how the behaviours currently called 'mental health' issues arise, from bad, damaged or threatening life contexts (Chapter 8; Johnstone & Boyle, 2018).

In future, those professing to be therapists and to be helping, must have a good knowledge of all the social, societal, economic, cultural, patriarchal, colonizing, and other life contexts which shape human behaviours. *This will require very different experiences and training* which is not based on 'learning the inner workings of the mind'. That learning has really been about learning how to manipulate words and social relationships, spinning, and engaging people for both good and bad, but it is no longer sufficient.

The plethora of therapies is an 'expert smokescreen'

There has always been a plethora of therapies claiming to be different, better than each other, and yet each 'authentic' (Chapters 2, 3 and 4. But we have seen that when examined more critically there is not so much difference between them (Chapters 3 and 4). There were four main conclusions from this, that:

- most of the 'differences' were only about how different therapists *talked* about what they do and why they think it works (Chapter 3)
- the practices themselves turn out to be quite similar once the theoretical assumptions are standardized and made concrete (Chapter 4; Frank, 1975)
- following the point above, a large part of the differences between therapies lay in how they managed to market and then *engage* with the people seeking help, and that these methods of engagement changed as new generations of people changed because new generations are shaped by different social, societal, and cultural contexts (requiring new 'therapies')
- there were many events which occur in almost all therapies which are likely to be useful and therapeutic, but which are never talked about as being therapeutic, since the marketing of therapies focuses on named differences in approaches, methods, etc., and are usually very abstract theoretical differences (Chapter 5)

The current therapies all use their specialized talking and engagement strategies to:

- form a working social relationship with a 'client' within a stranger/ contractual relationship
- be supportive and caring of them to some degree
- solve smaller or more localized conflicts in the client's life, which are amenable within an office
- act as a new audience to train new behaviours and skills where appropriate
- attempt to act as a new audience for them to change those thoughts and talking in ways that should be beneficial and reduce the suffering, especially for broader life conflicts

The first and last points account for the majority of differences between the many different varieties of therapy and how they market themselves. The rest is very similar and just differs in how it is talked about.

We need to do a more thorough analysis of language and how it works

As part of the first point, language has been taken for granted in this whole area as something originating inside a person which is an 'expression' of the (fictional) 'inner person looking out'. Changing this misleading metaphor is crucial because language is not only used for the majority of events in modern life to get things done (whether resources or social relationships), but also because (1) therapy itself now involves predominantly 'talking cures', (2) the behaviours shaped by living in bad life situations (the 'mental health' behaviours) are also predominantly about language, and (3) some of the most devastating behaviours shaped by living in bad life situations arise because people do not have functional 'discursive communities'; that is, people who listen and respond to them in 'normal' ways.

So, a lot rests on how we analyze and work to change our analyses of language both within therapy and outside.

'Therapy' needs to include a lot more

When 'mental health' behaviours are seen as responses to bad life situations and threats, there are more changes needed than encompassed by most approaches to psychotherapies and counselling. We can now look at Figure 10.1 which is based on the Figures of Chapter 8. More details of this will be given in Chapter 11.

'Treatment' 3. The 'treatment' type labelled as 3. is the mainstay of most current psychotherapies. The idea is to identify the behaviours which have emerged from bad life situations and then use rapport and 'therapeutic alliance' to stop those behaviours (Bourke, Barker, & Fornells-Ambrojo, 2021), increase other behaviours to replace them, or to change them in some other way. This applies to the majority of behaviours ('symptoms') identified in the DSM. Someone has recurring anxious thoughts and so the goal is to stop those thoughts occurring, to reduce them, or to replace them with 'nice' thoughts.

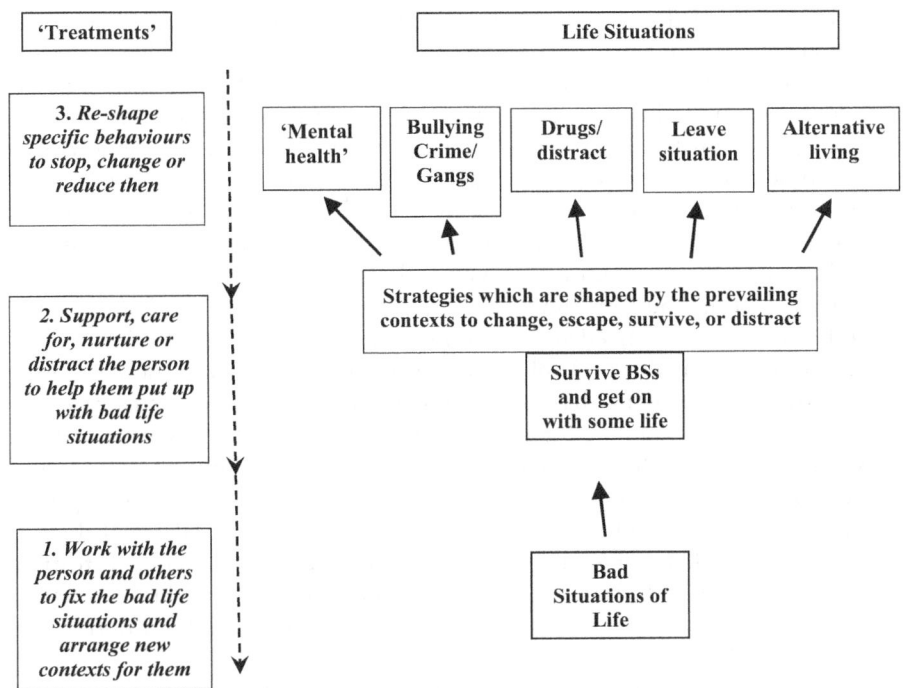

Figure 10.1 Three broad ways to help a person in distress

Therapists have become adept at this with all sorts of neoliberal-inspired exercises conducted (socially) with the therapist (note the marketing subtitles of these books: Chapman, Gratz, & Tull, 2011; Chen, 2019; Curran, 2013; Fox, 2015; Mullen, 2021; Raja, 2012; Riggenbach, 2013; Ruetter, 2019; Schwartz, 2010; Steven, 2020; Van Dijk, 2009).

These exercises can be successful, of course, but the problem is that there might only be a real and useful effect if the behaviours are *legacy behaviours* (behaviours shaped by bad life events but which remain even after those bad events and threats have ceased; Chapter 9). If the bad life situations are ongoing, the exercises are not likely to work or only work while in the presence of the therapist (which is partly what the marketing of the therapy stresses, as does the 'evidence base'). If the bad life situation is continuing, then the new or stopped behaviours will revert as soon as the person gets home (problems of 'relapse' are really problems of context). So, most of these sorts of therapies will only work if they are dealing with legacy behaviours.

'Treatment' 2. The second therapy approach is to just care for the person who is in a bad life situation and help them to put up with what is going on until other changes can occur. This is important to do in all circumstances, since the person will be suffering regardless. Unfortunately, professional requirements, especially for psychology-based therapies, do not encourage this (Chapter 2). Getting close to your 'clients' and hugging them, or taking them for coffee, is actively discouraged, and so such therapists are usually seen as aloof even when they are being effective. Building rapport and a therapeutic alliance is restricted only to very carefully pro-scribed professional and stranger-based events, even though the person is likely to need some raw care and might not have anyone else in their lives for this.

Other professions are better at caring for their recipients but are sometimes criticized for caring for the person without doing anything more substantial. We have seen that just putting up with bad life situations can allow for 'natural' changes to occur, but this should not be assumed (Chapter 9). Clearly, giving good care and love is needed but not in isolation.

Ironically, this is also probably what psychiatric medication is doing, slowing down the person hoping that some 'natural' changes might eventually be seen. The drugs typically slow people down and make them less aware, and hence less anxious', and if 'natural' changes do occur this can indeed be beneficial. But if nothing else is done then the drugs by themselves are not going to be helpful (and become unhelpful because of massive collateral effects of the drug intake and problems of withdrawal). The same applies to taking recreational drugs to 'put up with' the suffering of bad life situations and threats, they can be useful in relaxing the person in the short term but not useful if nothing else is changed (May & Quinn, 2021).

'Treatment' 1. Obviously, for this book so much more needs to be done in all forms of therapy to work at *directly stopping or changing the bad life situations and threats that are occurring* and which have shaped the behaviours labelled as 'mental health' issues. We saw in Chapter 3 that social workers are better at this, and the professional rules of most psychologists (Chapter 2) even prevent them from doing any of this ("That is someone else's job").

This needs to change. Perhaps this will not involve training psychologists to intervene themselves in people's bad life situations necessarily, but to work with some knowledge and in conjunction with other professionals and experi-enced carers. As mentioned above, there is no point doing your fancy CBT techniques 50 minutes a week if the person then returns to their house full of poverty and abuse until the following week's session.

An interesting point, which will be discussed more in Chapter 11, is that many of the bad life situations are society-created situations, such as patriarchal restrictions on life opportunities, poverty, racism, etc. But there is some evi-dence that just becoming aware that your bad life situation is not your own fault, or even your family's fault, but is shaped by the gross inequalities of modern societies, can in itself be 'therapeutic'. For women in feminist therapy, for example, they cannot smash the patriarchy overnight, nor quickly train their male partners to be perfect (who have their mates to contend with), but being aware that it is not you, but a bigger problem which has shaped your bad life situations, has been found to be helpful.

So, therapists need to develop their 'sociological imagination' and knowledge of the social, societal, economic, cultural, patriarchal, colonizing, and other life contexts which shape human behaviours, even when not being activists themselves (Guerin, 2016; Mills, 1959). And if governments really want to reduce the population statistics of 'mental health' issues, they need to bring about changes in the societal, economic, cultural, patriarchal, colonizing, and other life contexts which shape human behaviours.

References

Bourke, E., Barker, C., & Fornells-Ambrojo, M (2021). Systematic review and meta-analysis of therapeutic alliance, engagement, and outcome in psychological therapies for psychosis. *Psychology and Psychotherapy: Theory, Research, and Practice*, 94, 822–853.

Chapman, A. L., Gratz, K. L., & Tull, M. T. (2011). *The Dialectical Behavior Therapy skills workbook for anxiety: Breaking free from worry, panic, PTSD & other anxiety symptoms*. Oakland, CA: New Harbinger.

Chen, A. (2019). *The attachment theory workbook: Powerful tools to promote understanding, increase stability & build lasting relationships*. Emeryville, CA: Althea Press.

Curran, L. A. (2013). *101 trauma-informed interventions: Activities, exercises and assignments to move the client and therapy forward*. Eau Claire, WI: Premier Publishing and Media.

Fox, D. J. (2015). *Antisocial, borderline, narcissistic & histrionic workbook: Treatment strategies for Cluster B personality disorders*. Eau Claire, WI: PESI.

Frank, J. D. (1975). *Persuasion and healing: A comparative study of psychotherapy*. New York: Schocken Books.

Guerin, B. (2016). *How to rethink human behavior: A practical guide to social contextual analysis*. London: Routledge.

Guerin, B. (2020). *Turning mental health into social action*. London: Routledge.

Johnstone, L., Boyle, M., Cromby, J., Dillon, J., Harper, D., Kinderman, P., … Read, J. (2018). *The Power Threat Meaning Framework: Towards the identification of patterns in emotional distress, unusual experiences and troubled or troubling behaviour, as an alternative to functional psychiatric diagnosis*. Leicester, UK: British Psychological Society.

May R., & Quinn, K. (2021). Voice hearing and cannabis: A harm-reduction approach. In I. Parker, J. Schnackenberg, & M. Hopfenbeck, (Eds.), *The practical handbook of hearing voices: Therapeutic and creative approaches* (pp. 94–102). London: PCCS Books.

Mills, C. W. (1959). *The sociological imagination*. Oxford: Oxford University Press.

Mullen, M. (2021). *The Dialectical Behavior Therapy workbook for psychosis: Manage your emotions, reduce symptoms & get back to your life*. Oakland, CA: New Harbinger.

Raja, S. (2012). *Overcoming trauma and PTSD: A workbook integrating skills from ACT, DBT, and CBT*. Oakland, CA: New Harbinger.

Riggenbach, J. (2013). *The CBT toolbox: A workbook for clients and clinicians*. Eau Claire, WI: PESI.

Ruetter, K. (2019). *The Dialectical Behavior Therapy skills workbook for PTSD: Practical exercises for overcoming trauma & post-traumatic stress disorder*. Oakland, CA: New Harbinger.

Schwartz, A. (2010). *The complex PTSD workbook: A mind-body approach to regaining emotional control & becoming whole*. London: Sheldon Press.

Steven, R. F. (2020). *Psychosis recovery guide: A survivor's handbook to overcoming mental breakdown*. Published by author via Amazon.

Van Dijk, S. (2009). *The Dialectical Behavior Therapy skills workbook for bipolar disorder: Using DBT to regain control of your emotions and your life*. Oakland, CA: New Harbinger.

11 Reimagining 'treatments' in their social and societal contexts

What do we do instead?

After Chapters 1 to 10, it is time to start sketching what therapy needs to look like: how it needs to be reimagined. This is not about creating another in the long line of therapies with acronyms and fancy new theories and marketing. This is about reimagining the whole enterprise of therapy itself once we have rethought the whole notions of 'psychology' (Guerin, 2020a, 2020b) and 'mental health' (Guerin, 2017, 2020c). What develops is not a new therapy in that long line of therapies but a new and broader perspective on how to help and support people in distress.

Most of the therapy practices and thinking are shaped by having 'psychological' models

As summarized in Chapter 10, so many of the details of current therapies, as well as the broad justifications, only hold if you believe that there is an inside person or brain which originates and stores everything, and which needs fixing when things go wrong (Box 1.1). For example, with the mainstream models, to help a person with 'psychological problems' you only need a single expert in 'the human mind' to fix things because the problems to be fixed are 'in the mind'—people only need one therapist (although, in reality, people swap and change therapists all the time).

It is not just that most approaches to therapy derive from this, but that such models have also been used to justify for over a hundred years the governmental privileging of power to the medical profession to be able to 'read' and change' this 'inner person' or mind (Guerin, 2020c, Chapter 1). The inherent 'inside' secrecy of the (fictitious) 'psychological' models of human behaviour has perpetuated governmental control and the privileging of societally sanctioned 'experts in the human mind'.

The alternative way put forward of viewing such distress is that the person is having problems making their way in the world, and there is not something hidden 'deep' (whatever that means) inside the person somewhere that needs fixing. To solve these problems or at least to assist the person to find a way to deal with them or cope, requires many *different* sorts of changes and many cannot be solved by simply talking with a single person in an office, no matter how persuasive or tricky the therapist. For this definition, "The treatment of

DOI: 10.4324/9781003300571-14

mental or psychological disorders by psychological means", we also need to get rid of the phrase "by psychological means". This phrase means either it is based on thinking and secrets or it is based on language strategies (or both).

So, we need to do a thorough revision of the whole idea that people are determined by events originating inside of them, which they carry around inside, and which therefore need special practices and skills to 'reveal' and 'fix' so that only certain (government sanctioned) people can help. And as shown in Chapter 2 and Box 1.1, this involves almost every detail of what is currently taken for granted in therapy practices.

Reimagining the practices and thinking of therapy

I believe the whole idea that someone in distress 'needs some therapy' is false, along with 'having *a* therapist', certain ways of acting or talking being 'therapeutic', and the internecine disputes amongst 30 to 40 'different' forms of 'therapy' as to which works best. The whole image of current therapy is one of modernity: competitive with off-the-shelf solutions that fit all. And because they are only really different in the words they use, this plays out in abstract marketing claims and internecine disputes which cannot be resolved.

So, we really do not need the main features of traditional 'therapy' anymore. It was a way station predicated on the way the social relationships of modern society are formed and run, and on the neoliberal controls over the practices for governmental ends, which made use of the 'inside person' foundation (Guerin, 2020c; Chapter 1).

What we need to do for a distressed person, instead, is a contingent series of events which will usually involve several people. Even in the case of medicine for physical complaints we never just see one doctor: we have tests and imaging done by some, we have others to do surgery, and we have people to help care for us afterwards and rearrange our environments for best recovery and rehabilitation. We only ever imagined that we could 'see *a* therapist' and get well because the problems were attributed to forces 'inside' of us, and we were thought to be purely self-determining creatures with our 'minds' independent of external context, so we just had to make 'internal adjustments' (with a bit of specialized coaxing by 'your' therapist) in order to get well.

As another example, if the real problems for someone in distress are the conflicts and issues in their worlds, then a therapist needs to see that world, participate in it, experience the tensions for themselves, observe all the strategies and counterstrategies occurring (Tables 9.1 to 9.3), and show the person that their suffering is being taken seriously. Ever since the first contextual analyses by anthropology, it has been clear that alternative methodologies and procedures have been *necessary* for understanding humans because other methods assume you can just find out from or 'fix' whatever is in the person's head (Bohannan & van der Elst, 1998; Cubellis, 2020; Guerin, Leugi, & Thain, 2018). Figure 11.1 tries to show this using the format from Chapter 2. But current therapists are not trained in any of this.

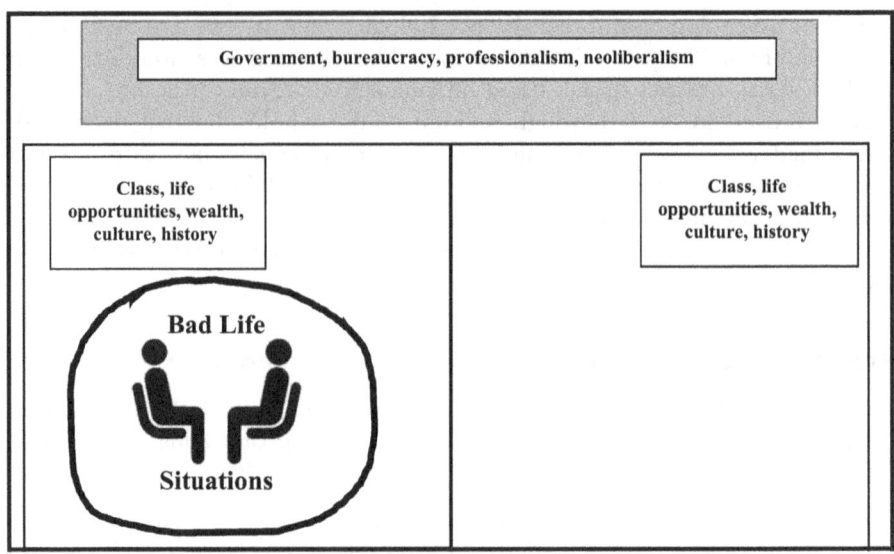

Figure 11.1 The 'therapist' engaging in and participating in the person's life world

This lack of connection or experience of a person's real-life world, other than what they selectively tell you in therapy sessions, has many other bad effects. Because the therapist is not seeing and participating in those environments the person is trying to negotiate in their life, this actually fuels the error of attributing casualty to fictions 'inside' the person (Chapter 1). If you cannot see what is shaping their behaviours, it gets attributed to something essential about them. As anthropologists and others who observe context know, only once you spend ample time with a person in their own world, do you truly begin to understand what is going on (Bohannan & van der Elst, 1998). And that includes possibilities of what you and the person might do to change things if they are suffering.

Following this, the lack of observation of context has also meant free rein for all the theorizing and marketing of therapies (Chapter 3). But all this needs to now stop. It was concluded that all this talk was just part of trying to *influence, suggest* or *persuade* the person to make the basic changes of current therapy (summarized in Chapter 10). These basic attempts have not changed over generations, but each generation has required new metaphors to be engaged so that these work: medical hypnosis for the socially obedient citizen who is still respectful towards doctors; CBT for the modern neoliberal working person; DBT for the confused adolescent who does not seem to respect authority, etc. What is done, however, is basically the same influence processes ('Treatment' 3. in Figure 10.1) which, as we will see, can still be helpful but is only part of the story of helping people who are suffering.

We need to stop 'peddling words' which make people think they are happier and that everything bad in their lives has been explained, and stop all the run-around word games in the therapy business. One of the main changes you come to when accepting this point is that while current therapies can certainly help, at least in some contexts, what they *name* as the crucial component, which goes hand-in-hand with their theories and marketing, is not likely to be the component event that leads to any change (Chapter 5). Box 5.1 listed many events that occur in almost all therapeutic situations, whatever the flavour or fad, which could be the real factor in change occurring (most likely this is never a single component anyway). However, I am not putting these forward as my 'new theory', they are just there to explore and use to think about idiosyncratic people in therapy and what is going on in their lives that might change. We have barely begun to explore these, partly because the verbiage and 'naming' of therapies as a market device has stopped any broader conceptualization of what might really be going on.

So, what do we need to do to support and help people in distress?

Figure 11.2 shows a rough schematic of a possible future for contextual help and support for people in distress. To start breaking up our complacency when thinking about therapies and healing, I go back to the broad model of 'mental health' given in Chapters 1 and 10, which includes a lot of behaviours shaped by living in bad life situations that are not generally called 'mental health' issues. From this we can see a minimum of at least three layers (as it were) of help or 'treatment' (Figure 10.1). They are simultaneous, however, and not sequential in any sense.

Beyond this broad outline, there are not going to be fixed rules, facts, theories or 'therapy hacks'. Everything must be sought through thorough contextual analyses including contextual observations, listening, and questioning. This extends the use of formulations and 'constructs' to explore more of the person's external world (Johnstone & Dallos, 2014). Each person will be different, and we would not expect to find any certainties that apply to everyone. We would expect to find patterns to be sure, and even common patterns, but always expect an exception with the person sitting in front of you, because they are bound to have slightly different contexts to all the others even if they superficially look the same. We do not need another DSM. If the purpose of the DSM was to put behaviours into categories, then every person will have their own combination shaped from their own idiosyncratic life situations. Everyone becomes their own DSM!

We can see some rough guidelines to guide the process of helping people who have had behaviours shaped in bad life situations and are suffering. This is shown in Figure 11.3.

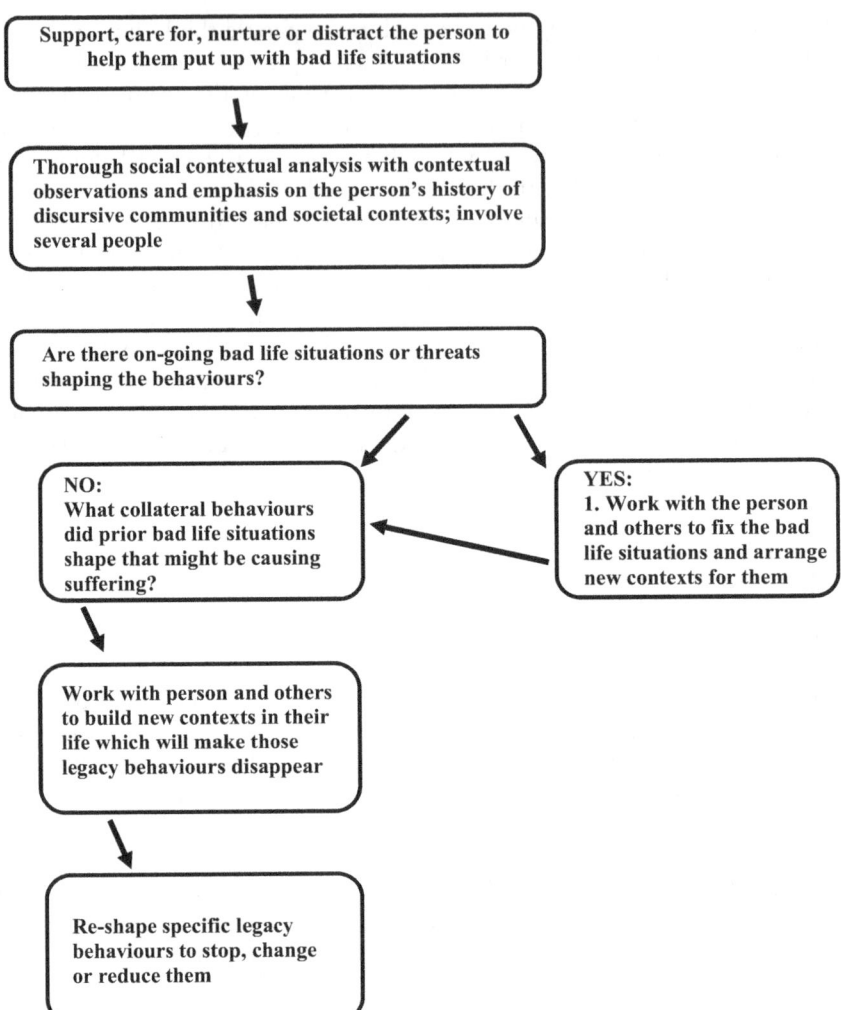

Figure 11.2 Rough schematic of a possible future for contextual help and support for people in distress

All my tables and boxes of contextual situations, strategies, and collateral effects, therefore, are merely *guidelines* to help *sensitize* you to the sorts of life strategies people get shaped into when trying to live in bad life contexts (Boxes 3.2, 4.1, 4.2, 5.1, 7.1, 7.2, 8.1, 8.2, 10.1; Tables 7.1, 7.2, 8.3, 9.1, 9.2, 9.3; Figures 9.2, 9.3; Guerin, 2020c, Chapter 4). The more experience you have with the huge range of contexts and strategies shaped in bad life situations, the more you will be sensitized and notice such patterns and know to ask about them.

Crisis	Care for the person humanely and give whatever support is needed Build social relationships with honestly and with whosoever the person wishes Let them tell their stories gradually Use Just Listening/ E-CPR/ etc. Move slowly into SCA/ formulations but only asking questions required for more story contexts **No** interrogation, questioning for therapist's ideas, interpretations, blame, over-medication
SCA/ Formulation	Discern the behaviours involved first, including other behaviours likely to be shaped or previously shaped (escape, distraction, criminal, other 'mental health' behaviours) Main question: What in the person's contexts has shaped these behaviours? Secondary question: What in the person's contexts has prevented alternative behaviours being shaped? Discern contexts for social relationships, discursive communities, cultural, opportunities, and societal barriers **No** interpretations or metaphors or categorizations, no DSM
Change life situations/ Threats	Directly change their bad life situations and threats Involve many people Involve people who have experience with those specific life situations Morph old situations into new ones Build new life situations with the person if needed Develop new discursive communities with the person (besides the therapist) **No** unilateral changes
Legacy behaviours	If the life situation is now liveable: CBT and other therapies to alter legacy behaviours in ways the person wishes **No** removal of the behaviours as they may still be useful in future life situations

Figure 11.3 Rough guidelines for 'therapy'

Support, care for, nurture or distract the person to help them put up with bad life situations

The first part is to just help people cope with the effects of bad life situations, giving social and resource support where needed. This form of helping does not explicitly aim to fix the person's behaviours or their bad life situation, but to 'keep them afloat', to help them 'put up with things' as well as possible until something changes or something else is done.

Such help is important for many reasons. First, of course, is the humanitarian aspect of just helping relieve someone's suffering when they are in trouble through no fault of their own. But we also saw in Chapters 4 and 9 that many 'mental health' issues are probably 'solved' by the passage of time, either through life situations naturally changing or new things happening in a person's life unrelated to any therapy. So, giving supportive help can sometimes help in this way, albeit a somewhat hit and miss approach.

In the case of young people, as an example, there is more hope for this because in most parts of the world, a lot of life contexts change anyway when beginning the adult years. Social relationships generally change, and social relationships are formed with new people outside the family, so 'natural changes' will often occur. But it is risky to assume this will take place, especially if the young person is in a very restrictive social context to begin with.

But the main drawback here is that raw support and caring is not going to be enough in most cases and waiting for 'natural' changes in life contexts is risky. Many therapeutic 'successes' might be due to 'natural' life context changes (cf. Lilienfeld, Ritschel, Lynn, Cautin, & Latzman, 2014). But if a therapy continues for over six months with nothing changing, clearly more needs to be done.

Oddly enough, as mentioned in Chapter 10, another form of support occasionally is the use of drugs prescribed by psychiatrists. Many of these can temporarily relieve some stress and anxiety and help people cope with some of their behaviours which have been shaped and give them a chance to find new changes in their life contexts. But only giving the medications with no other changes is not going to help, nor is continuing the drugs over a long period or upping the dose when no 'improvement' is seen. The problem here is that none of these drugs are cures—they do not solve people's bad life situations—and many become addictive and are difficult to stop safely (Guy, Davies, & Rizq, 2019; Moncrieff, 2019). Cures can *seem* to occur, but these are the result of gradual changes in a person's life situations over time unrelated to the medications. But in the meantime, the person is now in a new bad life situation since they might need one to two years to safely get off these drugs.

Giving unconditional support and care is also inhibited by governmental controls over current therapies, in two ways. First, social relationships with 'clients' are restricted in many ways so that normal human social reactions are not possible (Chapter 2). Second, the neoliberal character of modern therapies means that the therapist must be *seen* to be active and doing something to 'cure' the person or solve their problems. As we saw in Box 5.3, this leads to invasive questioning and gathering of mostly bureaucratic information in the initial period when care and support is probably needed. More recently, alternatives are being used (Bergström, Seikkula, Alakare, Mäki, Köngas-Saviaro, Taskila, Tolvanen, & Aaltonen, 2018; Browning & Waite, 2010; Guerin, Ball, & Ritchie, 2021; Myers, Collins-Pisano, Ferron, & Fortuna, 2021; Parker, Schnackenberg, & Hopfenbeck, 2021; Razzaque, 2019; Seikkula, 2020).

Thorough social contextual analysis with contextual observation and emphasis on the person's history of discursive communities and societal contexts; involve several people

A question that is frequently asked is: "What do we do without the DSM?" The question itself is very telling, from a discourse analysis point of view. The answer is simple to state but in practice it takes a lot more than just verbal questioning. The main thing is to do social contextual analyses of the person's behaviours and life situations, and especially of their 'discursive contextual history' (Guerin, 2016, 2017, 2020a, 2020b). This goes well beyond the normal demographic information questioning during the five minutes of rapport building, way beyond the focus on getting a diagnosis, and does a lot more than most formulations. Instead of categorizing the person into a DSM category, or trying to 'understand their mind' by telling fictional stories, we are trying to describe cooperatively what were the person's life contexts which shaped the behaviours presented as 'symptoms'.

I cannot give all the details here, but you and the person should end up with a good picture of the person's life contexts that includes the history and changes to getting resources, forming and maintaining social relationships, economic situations in a broad sense, patriarchal contexts, colonization contexts, opportunities available and blocked, and contexts specific to the idiosyncratic social relationships they have (cultural contexts). The point then is to look (with the person and others) at which of these contexts have been problematic, and how they have shaped the person's actions, talking, thinking and feelings (Guerin, 2020c). Then, being sensitized by life experiences and examples such as Tables 9.1 to 9.3, see how these have all interacted, with the life contexts shaping behaviours, which have then had collateral effects shaping further behaviours.

The story so far is somewhat general, but the basic procedures for doing all the above are there. From Chapters 7 and 8, we need to do the following, but these will occur through a range of people, not just one therapist, and be discussed with the person involved openly – as they are the expert here:

- fully listen to the person's stories of their lived experience (taking them seriously)
- find out if it is possible to participate in the person's life to any extent, to witness and experience yourself their bad life situations, as a social anthropologist would
- observe and inquire about the range of behaviours, looking for both 'non-mental health' behaviours (Figure 8.1) as well as multiple 'mental health' behaviours (Box 8.2), and do not limit your 'search' to a single one for use as a diagnosis
- observe and inquire about specific contexts which were in place, following Box 8.1; in most cases people have had other 'non-mental health' behaviours shaped at some point

- observe and inquire about specific 'mental health' contexts which were in place, following Figure 8.3; in most cases people have had more than one 'mental health' behaviour shaped at some point, so find out the contexts present when these appeared and disappeared
- observe and inquire about the contexts which made other solutions over time *not* possible (Figure 8.2; Guerin, 2020c, Chapters 4 to 8)
- look for the 'ordinary' origins of the behaviours and discuss the 'normal' functions of these with the person
- be cautious of too much questioning or inquiry, however, since sometimes this becomes yet another restrictive context for the person (like interrogation), and since many times the person *cannot* put into words their experience (and music, art, etc. might help here); make sure your questioning is to explore the person's own life and story context, not to satisfy your *own* administrative or theoretical leanings
- if the bad life situations have stopped, then explore how the legacy behaviours might have continued and gained importance (Tables 9.1 to 9.3)
- monitor your own language use and explanations and avoid abstractions, and try to stay with describing concrete observable behaviours and life situations
- where a lot of thinking, rumination or hearing voices is involved, explore the contexts which might have led to talking out loud being punished or reduced in other ways and the ways that not saying out loud changes our discourses (Tables 7.1 and 7.2)
- where there is a lot of emotional behaviours, explore which of the person's situations is too difficult to solve so there is no easy response they can make, or which situations cannot even be put into words (Box 7.2); again, avoid asking too many questions since the emotional behaviours indicate that they might not be able to put their events or experiences into words

There are two parts of describing life contexts that I will discuss a little bit more. This is because they are not normally noticed in everyday life (indeed they often work better for us if not noticed) and also because current therapists are not trained in these areas (primarily sociological and political analyses, and sociolinguistics and discourse analysis).

Societal contexts shaping human behaviour

While it is easy to observe and talk about the events shaped by our social relationships, whether good or bad, our behaviour is heavily shaped by the structures of our different societies and communities, but these are more difficult to observe and talk about. Many of these appear in our lives as limitations, barriers or unknown opportunities that are not available, and these are not enacted by a single person or even by people we know. All of this makes them difficult to observe and recognize as shaping our behaviours. For example, both males and females (cis) of all cultures are shaped into specific groups of behaviours that the others do not do, but this has been shaped by a multitude of different strangers mostly (including media) and not by a single, nameable individual (like if 'The Patriarch' was a real person). The differences can be stark, and both (cis) genders are shaped by this but in different ways (who must wear makeup and who refuses to wear makeup?). But the shaping of these behaviours is difficult to locate and observe even though very, very real.

This means that a lot of the societal, colonization, patriarchal, economic, and other 'sociological' contexts shaping our lives are not talked about and the behaviours are assumed to be 'decided' or 'chosen' by the individual inside their 'mind' (Chapter 1). However, if you are truly wanting to learn what shapes human behaviour so that you can assist people, then you need to know this because it accounts for a large part of our lives (e. g., Guerin, 2020b, 2020c).

This means that future 'therapists' need good training in recognizing and understanding these components of human behaviour. Once again, this training is not currently done when becoming a therapist because everything is assumed to originate 'inside' the person, and so you do not need to know all this (Box 1.1 and Chapter 2). Once more, the idea is not to have a single therapist who must have an extensive knowledge of everything, but they must be sensitized to notice and bring others in.

A final point for this and the discursive communities in the next section is that when societal imposed structures are shaping the 'symptoms (patriarchy, colonization, etc.; Fromene & Guerin, 2014), *the person will often be blaming themselves* since they, as well as everyone else, will not recognize that 'society' has really shaped their behaviours. This can be a clue for you.

Discursive communities shaping human talking and thinking

The other life context usually overlooked is the person's *history* of talking and getting things done through using language (Chapter 7), whether this is getting resources or maintaining social relationships (Guerin, 2016). I have stressed that those behaviours shaped by very restrictive bad life situations (formerly known as 'mental health' behaviours), are especially likely to result from living in life situations in which language does not have effects or is usually punished, and the person's 'words are broken'.

This means documenting the history and current situation with respect to the effects of the person using language (and not their linguistic competency, which is most often fine once they get into the right discursive contexts/ communities). This typically happens when trying to live in social relationships in which the person's words have been chronically punished, ignored, or opposed. Their words have no effects, and they are punished into a lot of silence and thinking. This is dangerous because most of what we get in modern life, all our resources and friendships and networks, is done through using language. Losing an effective language means losing a large part of life's outcomes and any future opportunities.

For the word (and, consequently, for a human being) there is nothing more terrible than a lack of response.

(Bakhtin, 1986, p. 127)

In this case, finding the discursive community history involves finding out the sorts of discourses they have used during their lives (directives, storytelling, gossip, arguments, blaming, joking and humour, conspiracy stories, etc.), and alongside this, finding out the contexts in which these discursive were said (usually their audiences) and the responses which typically occurred (silenced, responded with opposition or neglect, normal responses). "Did you ever get to tell stories about your day to your parents? What were their reactions?" "Did your parents joke around much with you?" Box 11.1 gives a more specific example.

Box 11.1 Questions for a person telling 'delusional' stories might be like these but include both historical and current discourses:

Who do you talk with normally in life?

What do you talk about?

Do have a lot of people to talk to or only few?

Do the people around you pay attention when you talk?

Do you have much success when you ask people to do things for you? Even simple things?

Do they do things you might ask them to do?

Do they enjoy your stories (not the delusional ones)?

When did the delusional stories begin and who were the listeners?

Do the delusional stories get people listening? Who? Friends? Family? Strangers?

Have the stories increased in length over time?

Have new parts to the story been added?

Do you tell exactly the same stories to everyone? Or change the stories slightly?

What happens when you tell other stories (what you did during the day, etc.)? Do people pay attention or not?

For people who have had damaging discursive communities in which little they said had any effect or outcome, it is crucial to find out these details, but the way of finding out more about their discursive and other contexts also needs some thought. The same applies to those who have no words for their experiences or have otherwise had talking heavily punished. Following on from Chapter 5, we just need to be careful not to blame them, ask 'why' questions, ask intrusive, unnecessary or personal questions, ask for details about what happened when they are reluctant, smooth over or minimize the effects of the incident, talk about your own experiences or other people's, interrupt with solutions or ideas or 'take over', take calls or get distracted, get angry on their behalf about someone else, promise everything will be okay, or jump straight into offering solutions or options.

You need to make sure the person feels heard first and begin to set up ways to have 'normal' effects of turn-taking in conversation (Guerin, Ball, & Ritchie, 2021). Tell them how what they say affects you (E-CPR), do tell them you are sorry this has happened to them, do tell them you will do what you can to help them, ask about their safety, and provide them with any information they request. Arrange your interactions so they can use language with safe but fruitful outcomes.

In all, therapeutic alliance is important (Bourke, Barker, & Fornells-Ambrojo, 2021), but we need to adjust it to different contexts. People who have had broken or damaged discursive communities in which their words have had little effect or only a punishing effect, need special consideration.

Are there ongoing bad life situations or threats shaping the behaviours?

At this point it should hopefully be clear whether the bad life situations or threats are either in the past or still current. The point of this whole approach (Figure 11.2) is that if there *are* ongoing bad situations then these need to be tackled rather than just try and stop or change the observed behaviours, since even if they change *in situ* within a therapy session, the behaviours will reoccur, or new ones will be shaped by the (current) bad life situations later on.

Given the hidden nature of some bad life situations (in which the person will often blame themselves), it is worth checking again the contextual analyses before going on, in case anything has been missed. As indicated earlier, this is especially so for societal contexts (such as effects of colonization or patriarchy), and for those who have lived in bad discursive communities. Remember Figures 9.2 and 9.3, where there are mixtures of current bad life situations, legacies from bad life situations which have now stopped, and collateral behaviours from all of these (although the full contextual analyses were not given).

Work with the person and others to fix the bad life situations or arrange new contexts for them

We no longer have an 'expert of the human mind' conducting therapy and fixing the person's inner world, but there are people who have long experience with different bad life situations and the behaviours shaped along with collateral effects, and these can be considered our new experts. They are experts in life's bad contexts and what happens when people try to survive in them. And just as a general practitioner might refer you to a physiotherapist and not do that work themselves, so we will in the future develop 'contextual experts' instead of 'experts of the human mind' or 'experts of DSM categories' (e. g., the 'anxiety specialist'). Most of these latter specialists will only appear (if at all) (see below) when considering ways to stop or change legacy behaviours.

Such 'contextual experts' will not necessarily have a university degree and sophisticated verbal knowledge, but they will have practical experience in particular bad life situations. So, depending upon the social contextual analysis, you might have the person spend time with financial planners with experience in the particular context (probably not someone from a bank), social workers, legal advice, women studies groups, women's shelters, former prisoners, family care workers, those who run decolonization workshops, peer workers who have lived in the same situations, a person experienced in family systems, etc. Some forms of family therapy and social work already do this, as well as some psychologists who do it 'behind the scenes'. This can be combined (as often happens already) with the first step of just supporting and caring for the person.

So, the good news from all this is that there are professionals, carers, and friends who are already helping people trying to survive in bad life situations, and we can pool all that expertise (along with other first-hand experiencers) to approach the difficulties of changing real life situations, since there will be similar occurrences whether we are dealing with 'mental health', crime, bullying, exit and distraction, drugs, etc. They will know far more of the strategies and outcomes which are shaped when living in bad life situations and go well beyond my limited Tables 9.1 to 9.3.

We might then see a new 'post-internal' form of relieving people's suffering, which does not differentiate between mental and non-mental health, and which uses common methods for changing the clients' external contexts, whether this is for verbal and other behaviours (since verbal is social). This *would not distinguish between* the expertise of first hand experiencers, and psychologists, social workers, psychiatrists, and other professionals, but instead distinguish between those who might specialize in common problematic contexts of modern life, common forms of social relationship conflicts, common bad contexts endured by women, common forms of conflict and suffering in Indigenous communities, or other specializations dictated by the external concerns giving rise to clients' suffering, and *not from* theoretical metaphors about 'inner' turmoil.

So, the future I envisage might be this: that people will have problems in their life situations and get trapped, and try to change these situations with normal behaviours, which then become chronic or distorted and lead to further problems and dysfunctions. To change these 'mental health' issues, however, we need *experts who specialize in the typical bad life situations* and how these lead (their functional relationships) to problems.

We no longer need specialists in general psychology or psychiatry or 'mind experts'

For example, if a young person has problems with drugs, then we do not need a generalized 'expert' in human behaviour or the mind, we need an expert in those bad life situations which shape drug problems in young people and how we can change those situations. This will involve someone with good participatory knowledge of the cultural, economic, and relationship problems based in a good understanding of modernity, rather than someone with general knowledge of an abstract human 'mind' or theories of cognition. Another good example is found in Durrant and White (1990).

At this point it is good to remind ourselves of Boxes 9.1 and 9.2. To change someone's behaviours we need to change the contexts which are shaping the behaviours; arrange new contexts which can shape the sorts of behaviours they want instead; include all the social, discursive and societal contexts of life, not just obvious parts of the physical environment; and change the available opportunities afforded by any life contexts (also compare Guerin, 1994, p. 76). Once we do this, the behaviours do not stop or get cured, they simply are no longer shaped and 'become irrelevant' or 'go into the background'. That is the nature of contextual changes, and we do not really want the behaviours to cease in all contexts because they might be useful one future day in a new context. This latter point is often said by first-hand experience people: that their anxiety or voice hearing has not stopped but been 'put in the background' as it were, and they often remark that they do *not* want those behaviours to completely leave forever. Anxiety and rumination, for example, are frequently useful and even necessary in planning for modern life.

How people's life contexts get changed is of course complex and idiosyncratic, and can include:

- changing the social relationships with people in their lives, meaning to change the resource-social relationship interactions or 'power' relationships (examples in some forms of family therapies; Guerin, 2020c, Chapter 5)
- removing the person (voluntarily of course) from their current life situations and providing whole new contexts for them (arranging a whole new life as Milton Erickson occasionally did, Haley, 1973)
- work with 'contextual experts' and the person to change specific life contexts to improve opportunities and make more alternative behaviours possible than they have had in the past (economic, patriarchal, colonizing, cultural, etc.)
- the above might need slow and careful setting up of new contexts and dealing with inherent collateral changes which occur, that could derail the process

Changing the societal contexts shaping human behaviour

I have already mentioned that we usually cannot easily see or change those patterns structured in our societies which shape our behaviours. We can, however, change the person's life contexts so they shape new behaviours not in line with society (although professional therapy associations do not relish this). This goes along with having people get involved in women's studies groups, decolonization groups, etc. (Smail, 2005; Guerin, 2020c). As mentioned earlier, while joining such groups and learning more about how society has shaped your behaviour does not stop society from still doing that, it does help in general.

In my view, learning about what has shaped your behaviours (contextual analyses) is frequently useful for alleviating suffering, even when little actually changes (see Chapter 3). Our research also frequently finds people reporting afterwards that doing the contextual analysis has helped them. It also can stop the person blaming themselves for their problems.

The other point to make about societal shaping of human behaviour is that the real problem is the presence of bad life situations in the first place. If governments and professionals were serious about reducing the growing rates of 'mental illness', then they should seriously work to reduce such situations happening in people's lives *in the first place* and put more money and resources towards that. Reducing the current gross inequalities in modern 'developed' societies would be the best way to reduce a range of societal issues, and 'mental health' would be one of those (Stiglitz, 2013; Wilkinson & Pickett, 2010).

Changing or building new discursive communities shaping human talking and thinking

I have already indicated earlier that analyzing discursive behaviours is difficult because the social shaping is not obvious. But if someone has had very poor responses to whatever they have said during their life, they are not likely to talk much (or talk delusions, extreme beliefs or 'word salad'). As outlined in Chapter 9, this usually increases what we call thinking, all the discourses we respond with but those not said out loud. People with damaged discursive communities will most likely have a distrust of talking out loud and do much talking not-out-loud.

To deal with this, we need experts in language strategies, not psychology. Much of sociolinguistics can be useful in showing how language and turn-taking normally works; although we do not want to set people up to merely to talk 'normally' but to also keep whatever creative and interesting discursive behaviours have been shaped under their unfortunate contexts (cf. Guerin, 2021). So clearly, from everything that has been written here, the way of repairing broken language is not to teach the person grammar or communication skills. Almost everyone has used language successfully in their life previously, so if you can get the right social/ discursive contexts for them, their functional language uses will happen again.

The point therefore is *to arrange things so they get successful social effects or outcomes for their talk*, and not just teach them to produce nice sentences which are polite (although polite sentences will often be more likely to get an effect that is positive and longer lasting). How this is done is highly variable and will depend on many idiosyncratic contexts about the particular person, their history of people responding to their talking, *and your own relationship to them*. The latter is often not considered, but is probably a component of most current therapies that are useful. I give merely suggestions below; use your own knowledge of your own social relationships and their history:

- Do not force them to always talk
- Do not assume they *can* talk about what is happening to them
- Just listen to them if they want to try talking and be very aware of how you respond
- Give authentic responses as far as this is possible (E-CPR i.e., what you really feel as a person when listening to them; it will not always be nice)
- If you are a therapist, remember that they know you know that you are mostly listening and responding because you are being paid, so do not pretend that this is not so
- Remember to ask them about, and listen to, what effects they see as coming from their different forms of talking
- Do not teach them talking skills or communication skills unless you find out that they never had these earlier in life (or they are younger)
- Remember that you are not teaching them about language; you are teaching them about social relationships and social exchanges and how these can be done in mutually beneficial ways by using language ("Use your words!")
- 'Teach' not in a didactic way but through how the two of you and others act and react
- Ask them about all the forms of talking and writing given above (and more) and focus on what those forms of discourse did for them, and what effects happened previously and now (part of finding their discursive contextual history)
- Most importantly, teach them about (re)forming and maintaining social relationships through social exchanges and reciprocity, in the varied contexts relevant to family, friends, and strangers
- Act as a new and genuine audience to them, knowing that your responding and social exchange will be the main factor that can help or hinder (or else dissociachotic responding will occur)
- Just doing this will begin to shape more useful language behaviours than they have had previously
- Work alongside them to find new, better audiences and learn how to differentiate these from their previous social relationships (a positive feature of my *Tree Hugging* and *Watching the Stars* therapies!)
- If the person wishes to continue in their current social relationships (which are not working), those other people will need to change in some way; how you do this as a therapist is difficult and most often ignored
- Read more yourself, and encourage the person if relevant, about sociolinguistics and discourse analysis to see what is good and usually functional in 'normal' conversations, and more importantly, always be aware that there are no generalizations, and all these suggestions and examples will only function in certain social, societal, cultural, discursive, economic,

patriarchal, colonized, and other life contexts; you need to adapt whatever you read to the current contexts

- Remember that part of the hidden benefits of *Tree Hugging* or *Watching the Stars* theories (Chapter 5), is that during all the 'incidental' things going on (travel, lunch, etc.) there are opportunities to use language and get decent and realistic outcomes from what you say; another disadvantage of highly controlled protocols of therapy dictated by 'professionalism'

The goal of all this is to get some new discursive communities for the person (or repair their old ones if this is still possible) in which normal language functioning will take place, such as listeners answering their questions, doing what they ask that is reasonable, listening to their stories and acting appropriately, being basically caring and interested, and responding with reciprocity and turn-taking (see socio-linguistics). But this is difficult because mainstream therapies often do not allow this because of professional rules (Chapter 2). Also, any 'authenticity' is often faked by therapists, but someone who has survived a broken discursive community all their life will be able to see right through this immediately. So, building or rebuilding discursive communities should be done slowly, piecemeal, and involve lots of other people, not just one therapist (Guerin, 2021).

What collateral behaviours did prior bad life situations shape that might be causing suffering?

If there is no current bad life situation (and you have rechecked carefully), then we are dealing with legacy behaviours which were shaped as collateral effects of earlier bad life situations. Tables 9.1 to 9.3 are mere starting point to discuss with the person, while including others with life experience as needed (peer workers, carers, professionals who also have experience).

The nature of those earlier bad life situations will suggest other people with more specific experience and expertise who might assist. For example, young people trapped (possible alternative behaviours are punished or prevented) in 'loving' middle-class families is a specific life situation that is common and shapes behaviours such as those labelled 'depression', self-harm, and 'eating disorders' (especially females who have other societal restrictions on their behaviours than do most males). But there are people who have extensive experience of living in these conditions and are now helping others. But self-harm and 'eating disorders' shaped in these conditions are going to need different ways of understanding and responding than the same superficially similar behaviours in another person's life context, and hence require other 'experts' (Westerman, 2021).

Work with person and others to build new contexts in their life which will make those legacy behaviours disappear

Once we have the legacy behaviours identified, the first step is to see whether these can be changed by changing things in the person's life contexts (as discussed in the section on changing or building new discursive communities shaping human talking and thinking). This is preferable, if possible, because it allows the 'problematic' behaviours to disappear while still being available should the context ever arise. New contexts can be built without having to focus on the 'problematic' behaviour itself, since 'focusing on the problem behaviour' is itself a social context which can have bad collateral effects.

As an example, for those with collateral 'speech disorders' or 'thought disorders' even when the original bad situations are gone, focusing on these to stop them has never been very successful, can shape new collateral behaviours, and can punish behaviours which might be useful in another context in the future. Likewise, trying to stop 'delusional talk' by persuading the person out of them has never been successful. Building new discursive communities with the person so they can get things done with their language without having to exaggerate storytelling is far safer. The delusional stories will just disappear.

Work with person and others to stop or reshape those legacy behaviours

Finally, we have all sorts of methods and techniques to change the behaviours being shaped by bad life situations, whether these behaviours are actions, talking, thinking, or feeling. We try to stop one person from having anxious thoughts, another from self-harming, another from taking drugs, another from committing crime, etc. These have been the mainstay of psychology (psychiatry focuses on giving drugs) and there are numerous versions of these (Chapters 3 and 4) and multiple 'activities' that might work (Chapter 10). Remember, though, that all these therapies have other component events occurring which might be the most useful part (Chapter 9).

Within the current 'mental health' realm, this sort of approach is done mainly by clinical psychologists, social workers, therapists, hypnotherapists, behaviour modification therapists, etc. Cognitive behaviour therapy was an attempt to bring together ways of changing people's actions as well as actions including talking and thinking. But they were brought together under a story that something was faulty or wrong inside the person and that the 'inside' behaviours (cognitions) needed to be stopped or changed.

My hope is that the best activities and components of these mainstream therapies will remain, but within Figure 11.2 they will only be a small part of assisting people who are suffering from living in bad life contexts. They have been straightjacketed by their own historical contexts and need to be more flexible and varied in their processes and ways of doing social relationships (Chapter 2). We need to enhance 'formulations' (Chapter 3) to include a person's whole social contextual and discursive contexts, and we no longer need the defective DSM categorization system, although various patterns might be found along the way (Guerin, 2020c, Chapter 4).

But primarily the major reimagining will be to assist people with observations of not just their behaviours but of their life contexts as well, and of working with the person to make changes to their contexts to change their behaviours. This reimagines the whole historical context of 'doing therapy', and this book only touches on some of the changes we might make to better assist people in the ways they want.

References

Bakhtin, M. M. (1986). *Speech genres & other late essays*. Austin, TX: University of Texas Press.

Bergström, T., Seikkula, J., Alakare, B., Mäki, P., Köngas-Saviaro, P., Taskila, J. J., Tolvanen, A., & Aaltonen, J. (2018). The family-oriented open dialogue approach in the treatment of first-episode psychosis: Nineteen-year outcomes. *Psychiatry Research*, 270, 168–175.

Bohannan, P., & van der Elst, D (1998). *Asking and listening: Ethnography as personal adaptation*. Long Grove, IL: Waveland Press.

Bourke, E., Barker, C., & Fornells-Ambrojo, M. (2021). Systematic review and meta-analysis of therapeutic alliance, engagement, and outcomes in psychological therapies for psychosis. *Psychology and Psychotherapy: Theory, Research and Practice*, 94, 822–853.

Browning, S., & Waite, R. (2010). The gift of listening: JUST listening strategies. *Nursing Forum*, 45, 150–158.

Cubellis, L. (2020). Sympathetic care. *Cultural Anthropology*, 35, 14–22.

Durrant, M., & White, C. (1990). *Ideas for therapy with sexual abuse*. Adelaide, South Australia: Dulwich Centre.

Fromene, R., & Guerin, B. (2014). Talking to Australian Indigenous clients with Borderline Personality Disorder labels: Finding the context behind the diagnosis. *The Psychological Record*, 64, 569–579.

Guerin, B. (1994). *Analyzing social behavior: Behavior analysis and the social sciences*. Reno, Nevada: Context Press.

Guerin, B. (2016). *How to rethink human behavior: A practical guide to social contextual analysis*. London: Routledge.

Guerin, B. (2017). *How to rethink mental illness: The human contexts behind the labels*. London: Routledge.

Guerin, B. (2020a). *Turning psychology into social contextual analysis*. London: Routledge.

Guerin, B. (2020b). *Turning psychology into a social science*. London: Routledge.

Guerin, B. (2020c). *Turning mental health into social action*. London: Routledge.

Guerin, B. (2021). Contextualizing 'psychosis' behaviors and what to do about them. In *Towards a paradigm shift: Clinical cases in psychosis. Hacia un cambio de paradigmas: Casos clinicos en psicosis* [Dual language publication]. Madrid: Ediciones Psara.

Guerin, B., Ball, M., & Ritchie, R. (2021). *Therapy in the absence of psychopathology and neoliberalism*. University of South Australia: Unpublished paper.

Guerin, B., Leugi, G. B., & Thain, A. (2018). Attempting to overcome problems shared by both qualitative and quantitative methodologies: Two hybrid procedures to encourage diverse research. *The Australian Community Psychologist*, 29, 74–90.

Guy, A., Davies, J., & Rizq, R. (Eds.) (2019). *Guidance for psychological therapists: Enabling conversations with clients taking or withdrawing from prescribed psychiatric drugs*. London: APPG for Prescribed Drug Dependence.

Haley, J. (1973). *Uncommon therapy: The psychiatric techniques of Milton H. Erickson, M. D.* New York: Norton.

Johnstone, L., & Dallos, R. (Eds.). (2014). *Formulation in psychology and psychotherapy.* London: Routledge.

Lilienfeld, S. O., Ritschel, L. A., Lynn, S. J., Cautin, R. L., & Latzman, R. D. (2014). Why ineffective psychotherapies appear to work: A taxonomy of causes of spurious therapeutic effectiveness. *Perspectives on Psychological Science*, 9, 355–387.

Moncrieff, J. (2019). *A straight talking introduction to psychiatric drugs (Second edition): The truth about how they work and how to come off them.* London: PCCS Publishing.

Myers, A. L., Collins-Pisano, C., Ferron, J. C., & Fortuna, K. L. (2021). Feasibility and preliminary effectiveness of a peer-developed and virtually delivered community mental health training program (Emotional CPR): Pre-Post study. *Journal of Participatory Medicine*, 13, 1–11.

Parker, I., Schnackenberg, J., & Hopfenbeck, M. (Eds.) (2021). *The practical handbook of hearing voices: Therapeutic and creative approaches.* London: PCCS Books.

Razzaque, R. (2019). *Dialogical psychiatry: A handbook for the teaching & practice of Open Dialogue.* London: Omni House Press.

Seikkula, J. (2020). From research on dialogical practice to dialogical research: Open Dialogue is based on a continuous scientific analysis. *Systemic Research in Individual, Couple, and Family Therapy and Counseling*, 7, 143–164.

Smail, D. (2005). *Power, interest and psychology: Elements of a Social Materialist understanding of distress.* London: PCCS Books.

Stiglitz, J. E. (2013). *The price of inequality.* London: Penguin.

Westerman, T. (2021). Culture-bound syndromes in Aboriginal Australian population. *Clinical Psychologist*, 25, 19–35.

Wilkinson, R., & Pickett, K. (2010). *The spirit level: Why greater equality makes societies stronger.* New York: Bloomsbury Press.

Index

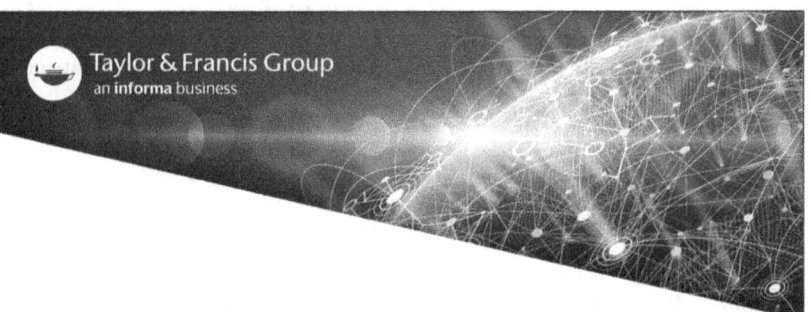

Taylor & Francis Group
an **informa** business

Taylor & Francis eBooks

www.taylorfrancis.com

A single destination for eBooks from Taylor & Francis
with increased functionality and an improved user
experience to meet the needs of our customers.

90,000+ eBooks of award-winning academic content in
Humanities, Social Science, Science, Technology, Engineering,
and Medical written by a global network of editors and authors.

TAYLOR & FRANCIS EBOOKS OFFERS:

A streamlined
experience for
our library
customers

A single point
of discovery
for all of our
eBook content

Improved
search and
discovery of
content at both
book and
chapter level

REQUEST A FREE TRIAL
support@taylorfrancis.com

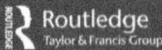
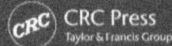